DYSLEXIA

Problems
of Reading
Disabilities

DYSLEXIA
Problems
of Reading
Disabilities

Herman K. Goldberg, M.D.

Associate Professor of Ophthalmology, Wilmer Institute, The Johns Hopkins Hospital; Associate Professor of Pediatrics, The Johns Hopkins Hospital; Chief of Ophthalmology, Kennedy Institute, The Johns Hopkins Hospital; Director, Division of Ophthalmology, Sinai Hospital of Baltimore; Chief of Ophthalmology, The Good Samaritan Hospital, Baltimore, Maryland

and

Gilbert B. Schiffman, Ed.D.

Director, Division of Education, Evening College and Summer School, The Johns Hopkins University; Associate Professor of Education, Evening College and Summer School, The Johns Hopkins University; Assistant Professor of Special Education, Department of Pediatrics, The Johns Hopkins University, Baltimore, Maryland

GRUNE & STRATTON
New York and London

Library of Congress Cataloging in Publication Data

Goldberg, Herman K
  Dyslexia.

  Bibliography: p.
  1. Dyslexia. 2. Communicative disorders in
children. I. Schiffman, Gilbert, joint author.
II. Title. [DNLM: 1. Dyslexia. WL 340 G618d 1972]
RJ496.A5G65   616.8'553   72-8139
ISBN 0-8089-0784-0

Grune & Stratton, Inc.
111 Fifth Avenue
New York, New York 10003

Library of Congress Catalog Card Number 72-8139
International Standard Book Number 0-8089-0784-0
Printed in the United States of America

Dedicated to

CECE, HARRY, and BARBIE

Contents

Foreword

In this era of unprecedented publication explosion there is hardly a topic in any area of human interest that has not been seized upon by the printing press. Articles by the tens of thousands, monographs and books by the countless dozens are foisted on the reading public in an unending flow brought out in scientific and lay journals, in volumes by single authors, in symposia and edited tomes with a host of contributors.

The problem of dyslexia did not fail to share this fate. An issue virtually unknown to the general public before 1917, when Hinshelwood brought out his book on Congenital Word Blindness, has resulted in an astronomical effusion which, if assembled together, could easily fill many shelves of a large special library. There has been an avalanche of varieties of nomenclature, etiological theories, therapeutic thou-shalts and thou-shalt-nots, serious research studies, good-will sermons and just plain verbiage.

As one who has lived through this development from its beginning, I have witnessed pontifical assertions of a genetic origin, pseudoneurological edicts about conflict of cerebral dominance, pseudodynamic reference to psychoanalytic principles, and variegated educational groping.

This is not to say that important work has not been done and reported. Concerned people in the fields of education, neurology, psychology, psychiatry, and ophthalmology have done their best to become acquainted with the study, understanding, and remedy of the difficulty and its ramifications. However, there has been a remarkable dearth of intercommunication so that we are still confronted with the spectacle of the different disciplines working in isolation, sometimes finding themselves somnambulating in each others' camps.

For this reason it is refreshing to come upon a valiant effort to pull all the factual knowledge obtained so far together and to integrate the various fragments into a substantial edifice centering upon the one thing that is common to all the building stones namely, the individual child who is the victim of the difficulty and needs primary consideration.

Dr. Herman K. Goldberg, an outstanding ophthalmologist who from an early time has given earnest attention to children and their reading disabilities, has made himself thoroughly familiar with all the aspects of the problem. He has managed to gather up all the clusters and putting them together under one roof in which the pertinent disciplines are linked together with interconnecting doors. He has done so with an astute ability to pick out the scientifically established facts without espousing any unproven hypothesis and tradition but instead coordinating solid, indisputable data from the areas of early predictability, psychology and psychological evaluation, neurological considerations, visual and auditory factors, psychiatric implications, and biochemical investigations. Such an undertaking has been long overdo. While this accentuates the complexity of the problem, it nevertheless works at the same time toward a welcome clarification.

Dr. Goldberg, who in his medical setting has not himself had any teaching experience with dyslexic children, has had the profound wisdom to invite and receive the collaboration of Dr. Gilbert B. Schiffman, nationally prominent educator who, as part of his universal pedagogic interests, has given a great deal of attention to the problems of dyslexia. He is the author of the chapter on Education in which his authoritative familiarity with the situation rings through every sentence. He not only, to use the vernacular, tells it as it is but presents an excellent plea for its ideal amelioration, with a heartwarming dedication to the dyslexic child, his family, and his teachers.

This is a book which can be of considerable use to everyone in any way concerned with children's reading, be he (or she) an educator, psychiatrist, psychologist, pediatrician, family physician, ophthalmologist, or a sufficiently educated parent.

Having had four decades of contact with children and their many problems, including dyslexia, I can say that I enjoyed reading this book and profited from it.

LEO KANNER, M.D.
Professor Emeritus of Child Psychiatry
and Honorary Consultant,
The Johns Hopkins University School of Medicine

Preface

The field of education has long needed a text that relates the medical disciplines to education. This publication attempts to fill that need. The necessity of recognizing the contributions from many disciplines is important, but it is difficult to relate these medical contributions to areas of learning in a simple and uncomplicated manner. Twenty years of close contact with teachers and administrators have provided an opportunity to understand the areas in which the problem of the retarded reader and of the educator can best be assisted by medical intervention.

The publication of this book also provides us with the opportunity to express to numerous colleagues our sincerest gratitude for sharing with us over the years their knowledge in the areas of their specialization. To Dr. Robert E. Cooke, for his encouragement and guidance in bridging the controversial gaps involved in the many aspects of learning. To Dr. Leo Kanner, Dr. Henry Mark, Dr. Katrina DeHirsch, Dr. Jeannette Jansky, and Dr. Paul Leand for sharing with us their knowledge so that we might be able to provide a distillation of their expertise in organizing our concepts of the many etiological factors that cause a reading disability. Acknowledgment is also made of the assistance of Dr. David Vess, whose efforts were important in the completion of this volume.

H.K.G.
G.B.S.

PROLOGUE: A CASE HISTORY

*On September 7, 1968, a letter from a distressed parent gave the
following information about her son:*

Charles was born July 26, 1953. His birth was
an assisted breech delivery. He was examined by
a pediatrician and general practitioner and found
to be in good health despite the breech delivery.

He was an excellent baby, slept well, and took
his formula well, crying only when hungry or wet.
His changeover from formula to solid foods was not
satisfactory. He crawled at 5½ months and walked
at 11 months. He was riding a tricycle before his
second birthday. He did not speak until age 2½,
or perhaps 2¾, and then spoke sentences.

At one-and-a-half years he fell down a flight of
stairs in our apartment. He had tried to walk down
backwards and lost his balance. He lay on the floor
below until I picked him up. I put him into his
crib, and when he dozed off he was immediately
awakened. His doctor was called and came to the
house. He found nothing wrong with the baby.

At age two he climbed to the top of a sliding
pond; when he reached the top he lost his balance
and went over, flying through the air, landing on
the ground alongside the sliding pond. The ground,

1

while dirt, was solidly packed. He cried, but when
I picked him up and comforted him, he walked
home. By afternoon, he had calmed down enough
to go outside and play.

He was a good child, very attractive looking,
but he could not defend himself against the aggressive children in the garden apartment where we
lived. We constantly were forced to talk to our
neighbors about their children hitting Charles.
When we moved to our own home, Charles unable
to fight back in order to protect himself, would
often take the nearest object, perhaps a toy, and
throw it, becoming unpopular with some of the
neighborhood mothers.

He entered kindergarten at age 5. In May of his
first school year, I was called to school for the
usual school conference. The teacher told me
Charles refused to finger-paint and draw, that he
only wanted to build with blocks. She had asked
the school psychologist to observe him. He found
Charles to be bright and when I asked for a
detailed examination, I was told they wouldn't
have the time to see him until the next year.
I discussed the interview with my husband and we
decided to have private testing. The psychologist
found Charles to be bright and cooperative. His
Stanford-Binet scores were between 115 and 120.
He was found to have small-muscle coordination
problems and had not selected which hand to use.

I discussed his findings with the kindergarten
teacher. The principal then decided to retain him in
kindergarten, saying he was not reading-ready.
The psychologist we had engaged went to see the
school psychologist and principal. After he went
over the test scores, they agreed to promote him to
Grade 1. He entered Grade 1 at age six. He was
not learning to read, and we were pressured to take
him for an electroencephlogram. We took him to
the Neuropsychiatric Center for a complete neuro-

logical exam and they found everything in the
normal range.

The pressure at school was building up and
Charles became so upset he continually ran to the
bathroom. The center decided it was an emotional
problem and agreed with the school that he repeat
first grade. He did not learn to read after being
retained in the first grade. In the meantime, we
went to a private psychiatrist. Charles was his
patient for 2½ years; they got along beautifully.
He became the most well adjusted nonreader. Dr. A,
the psychiatrist discharged him with the earth-
shattering remark, "I've taken him as far as I can.
I don't know why he's not reading, it must be a
developmental lag."

While Charles was going to Dr. A, we engaged
remedial reading tutors to work with him, with
very little success. In order to do something more
constructive for my son, I secured a part-time job.
As soon as I had saved a little money, I took him
to the university reading clinic for evaluation.
Dr. B, a clinical psychologist and assistant to the
director of the reading clinic, evaluated him.
He found his attention span poor and his reading
low enough for him to be called a nonreader.
He was then in Grade 2, age 8½. He suggested we
go to Dr. C in the city, to look into the possibility
of his taking vision training. Before going to Dr. C
we took our son to Dr. D, an ophthalmologist
connected with the Orthoptic Training Clinic at the
hospital. He found nothing wrong with our son's
eyes and told us to look for an answer to his reading problem elsewhere. After discussing the inci-
dent with Dr. B, we decided to follow his advice
and visit Dr. C. Dr. C had recently been appointed
to a committee on dyslexia. After seeing him twice,
we were sent home to do various optometric
procedures. This was in June, 1962. In September
1962, Charles was accepted for intensive office
work twice a week. We still continued to do home

procedures. He was discharged a year later. For a
number of years we returned for reexaminations
and they showed that Charles was maintaining his
gains. His attention span had improved, but his
reading gains were small.

While going to Dr. C, Charles also went to
Dr. E at the university. For a nine-year-old boy, he
had a busy schedule. All day he went to school
and at 3:30 we started all over again. Two days a
week he went to Dr. C, two day a week to the
reading clinic, and once a week to Dr. E. We
received no help from any government agency or
our school district. My husband is in state service
and, financially, the going was most difficult. In the
meantime, more pressure was being placed on us
as parents by the school principal. She wanted
another neurological examination and tried to
pressure us to put our child into private school.
Disgusted, I went to see our family pediatrician.
He suggested we go to see Dr. F, a pediatric
neurologist. He found Charles to be a bright boy
who had a reading problem called dyslexia. He told
us not to place our son in the county-run special
classes or in any other private school. In a tele-
phone conversation with our school psychologist,
he told him to stop harassing us. The school
superintendent then decided to transfer Charles to
another elementary school, with a more sympathetic principal. Charles was then 10½ years old.

During his ninth year, Charles attended the
reading clinic for four private sessions. His reading
went up to the 2.1 grade level. With the transfer
in mid-year to a new elementary school, he went
down to 1.7 in his reading. He was then in fourth
grade and receiving reading help, in a group situation, by the school's reading specialist. I decided
to withdraw him from our school district. I
enrolled him in the day school of the university
reading institute. He was then in fifth grade, age 11.
Despite intensive class work, he only made a two-

month reading gain. It was decided that he needed
one-to-one reading help, and they would not
continue to keep him in school. He refused to
return to the neighborhood school. In desperation
I called Dr. X and he recommended the Country
Day School. Charles attended it for one-and-a-half
years. It was a school for slow learners and
created more problems then it cured. They gave
him no remedial reading, and many of the children
had severe emotional problems. In desperation
I went to see an educational therapist. She is
presently the director of a perceptual motor project
funded by the federal government. As a graduate
of the Institute, she programmed Charles in all the
exercises. Her friend, a reading specialist, worked
diligently in the reading and handwriting area. His
handwriting improved, but not the reading. Later
we were sent to the Institute to see Dr. G. We
worked seven days a week. It was a most trying
period in both our lives. He was officially on the
program for two years, and continued the exercises unofficially for one year. The years were
quickly passing by. Charles was almost 13 and he
was returning to the neighborhood junior high
school. They insisted on new test data. I had him
tested in the spring of 1966 at a research and
evaluation center. They could not understand why
his reading gains were so small and claimed his
perceptual problem was not that bad. They also
threw in a remark for good measure, "Maybe he
has a tumor growing in his brain." In the summer
of 1966, he was examined by Dr. H at the Children's
Mental Health Clinic. He found no brain tumor
but "severe central nervous system dysfunction."
    In the summer of 1966, he also was given
vision and tachistoscopic training and worked very
diligently. He made no reading gains. The exercises were given by a noted reading authority who
is quoted continually in the literature. It is my
feeling that reading must be taught carefully not

by machines but by well-trained teachers.

Last year he complained about his eyes tearing. I was reluctant to go to an ophthalmologist because previously (at age 6½ and 8½) he had been examined, and nothing wrong was found. I finally took him to see an ophthalmologist whose son had dyslexia. I felt he would give me an honest appraisal of the situation. He found that Charles had a convergence problem of 30 diopters. He sent us for a work-up to the Dyslexia Laboratory. He was seen by a doctor who recommended surgery, but he would not tell us whether it would help his reading. Our son is now 15½ years old, he is well liked by his teachers and is maintaining above-average grades. He has been through so much during his young life that I feel complete honesty is necessary so that he can make the choice of whether to have surgery or not. His reading teacher has told him he needs eye muscle surgery. We are faced with a most difficult decision if surgery is necessary. Your guidance and recommendations are desperately needed.

CASE STUDY

When seen in consultation, the abundance of evaluations was impressive. Among the reports was a transcript of the obstetrician's delivery of the patient, an EEG report, a report of a college reading center which included psychological, audiometric, and visual examinations, an educational evaluation, and recommendations for remediation. He had been seen by a developmental optometrist who treated him for 2 years with a visual training program, at the end of which he stated that "Charles was now able to respond to reading instruction at the appropriate level." Then he was seen by a pediatrician who wrote that "in spite of his reading disability, Charles should take his place in society as a productive member. He must function with youngsters who except for reading ability, are his peers." He was seen and treated for three years by advocates of, and with methods of, neurological organization.

One year later the child was taken to another reading center, which stated: "His case is a mild one compared to many we have solved here.

This is what we are trained and prepared to do to an extent which does not exist in any other organization." He was then seen by another developmental optometrist who treated him with eye exercises. After another 2 years the child was taken to another reading center for further evaluation. Finally, eye surgery was suggested. Consultation with other ophthalmologists negated the need or value of this procedure and no surgery was done. The child developed a great interest in sailing and, now being age 17, he expressed a desire to enter the maritime service. His grades began to improve under no special remedial therapy except that provided by the public schools. He received one A and four B's and an award of Honorable Mention for Academic Achievement.

On arrival for consultation, the following status was obtained: Findings at this time follow: full-scale IQ 112, but with a range of abilities from IQ of 45 to 112 or a range from the trainable-retarded to a bright average. The performance evaluation varied from 74 to 108, IQ equivalent scores. The verbal scores also showed a great variation of 45 to 112. The low score suggested an auditory handicap which, when once circumvented, allowed him to function at a normal level. His ocular examination showed an intermittent exotropia of 20 prism dioptres, but with normal near-point convergence and good retinal correspondence. No surgery was recommended.

In view of his good recent academic progress, and his specific handicaps, Charles was encouraged as to his future ambitions and the parents were counseled as to the avoidance of undue pressures. One year later, a note came from another ophthalmologist who wrote that the parents had seen him with a further request for ocular surgery to cure his dyslexia.

This case again demonstrates that it is a fine line that determines the pressures that should be

exerted and where parents and teachers should
cease to exercise their aggressions. Twelve years
after, this parent is still looking for a magic
panacea (in this case muscle surgery) to cure her
son's difficulties in the area of reading.

This case emphasizes the complexity of
dyslexia, its enigmatic aspects and the frustration
of parent and child involved in such a problem.
This child at one time or another has been brought
to every professional discipline of the dyslexia
spectrum for evaluation and therapy. It is questionable which, if any, had an effect on the natural
evolution of the problem. What appears in the
parents written history as a total devotion to
seeking the solution of the problem might, in
reality, have been 15 years devoted to an aggra-
vation of the problem.

Introduction to the Reading Problem

This book is about children who are underachieving in reading and other language skills. There are many reasons why these children have difficulties. Some of these children have no known physical disability and their underachievement is not commensurate with a lack of potential. This is an attempt to explore those factors that are related to the child's failure to achieve his total potential.

The ability to read is probably more important today than at any other time in history. For centuries, when reading was not essential to an agrarian livelihood, this ability meant primarily an enhanced social and economic status in society for a very few people. With the rise of vernacular languages, the invention of the printing press, and urbanization and industrialization, the ability to read gradually became an imperative need for great numbers of people. As the modern world developed, its scientific discoveries and communicative innovations, its intellectual controversies and multiplying literary output, and its demand for popular education produced strong pressures for more people to read more printed material than ever before.

Certainly, ours is the most rapidly changing era in history. As science and modern technology continue to shrink our world ever smaller and to search into space for new worlds to explore and describe, our lives become forced into more and more complicated patterns. The pace of this veritable explosion of knowledge is breathtaking. Most of us like to read for relaxation and enjoyment and for the satisfaction of being well-read persons. "Keeping up" demands of an individual the accumulation of more knowledge than has ever been necessary before, and it taxes our ability to interpret written material more than do almost any of our other abilities. A truly vast amount of reading is now required, not just to be well-read, but to maintain one's proficiency in one's work and to try to solve the perplexing problems of modern living.

In 1877 Kussmaul[1] called attention to a phenomenon which he called "word blindness." He referred to a patient who was unable to read although his vision, intellect, and speech were unimpaired. In 1896, Morgan[2] published the case of a normally intelligent boy who had great difficulty in learning the letters of the alphabet; only with the greatest effort could he spell out monosyllabic words, and the impact of the words seemed to convey no impression to his mind. There was no impairment of his arithmetic abilities. Morgan's report was the first which was not associated with a history of neurologic problems. Hinshelwood in 1917 defined the condition as one in which an individual with normal vision (and therefore seeing the words distinctly) is no longer able to interpret written and printed language.

There have been other reports of similar cases; gradually, the condition, originally called alexia, has been termed *dyslexia*, and, more recently, as a specific learning disability. Larger groups of children have been termed "dyslexic" who might well be included in the low educable category. The heterogeneity of students who manifest learning disabilities has made identification and treatment more complex because we are not always talking about the same type of child.

Orton[3] designated dyslexic children as a group including those who are retarded in reading much below their achievement in other subjects, whose attempts at reading are characterized by frequent reversals and by confusion between words such as *saw* and *was*, and who show a greater facility in mirror reading than do normal readers. The frequency of reversals caused Orton to suggest the word *strephosymbolia*, meaning twisted symbol.

The principal criteria of this group of cases are these:

1. The reading disability is specific. The acquisition of reading skill lags behind the other scholastic achievements, and reading does not measure up to expectations normally justified in conjunction with the child's psychometric test age.

2. There is a tendency to reverse letters and words. Many children normally reverse- or mirror-write in the first and second grade. The average reader soon corrects this abnormality, but the reader who has a specific defect retains these characteristics.

3. The confusion extends over all of reading. In some cases the child may spell the words correctly but is unable to read them, or he may show a complete disability in spelling as well as difficulty in reading. Some children substitute other words for those they cannot read. Some of the children are especially adept at looking at a picture and making up their own story while pretending to read from the text.

In this day of emphasis upon universal education, the critical importance of the ability to read well, and with comprehension, becomes clearer when we realize that during the later school years almost ninety percent of a student's studies depend directly upon his reading ability. The student who fails to develop a highly skilled reading ability is faced with a serious handicap in his future as a productive citizen of the world. The more obvious disadvantages of being a poor reader include failure in school, the prospect of a less rewarding job, lower lifetime earnings, less social status, and fewer of the many things commonly associated with happiness and success in our society. Such an individual, robbed of the richness and fullness of life that is to be gained through reading literature, poetry, history, and philosophy, can never be expected to contribute to society to his fullest capacity.

Unfortunately, the reading problem has been found to be associated also with far more serious consequences for those whom it plagues. The problems inevitably interwoven with reading failures—seemingly the causes of poor reading or the results of it—may lead to juvenile delinquency and other dangerous antisocial consequences.[4] Almost without exception, children who are delinquent or considered to be "problem children," are below average levels in reading ability. Many educators

have concluded that nonreading is an early symptom of anta-
gonism and aggression against discipline and authority. The
frustrated nonreader rebels; as he falls further behind in reading, he becomes even more disturbed and antisocial. This growing inadequacy makes it difficult for him to participate in the
regular classroom situation, and his increasing alienation from
his own peer group may lead to continued failure and possible
future misconduct.[5]

Within the past five years, reading retardation has become
a really pressing question. Two UNESCO meetings and a State
Department conference are among the hundreds of sessions
which have been held to discuss the subject. Presidential and
governmental commissions have been organized. Several million words have been written. Animated groups discuss the
problem whenever educators meet. There is much to talk about.
It is estimated that 20%–40% of our school population is handicapped by reading problems. There may be as many as 8,000,000
to 20,000,000 of our school population who have reading
problems.

A renewed and widespread interest in dyslexia is making
itself felt even among those who have never used the term
before. Although dyslexia tends to be an ambiguous term,
"reading" itself is a term of great ambiguity. It is little wonder
that research studies and the literature are subject to contradictory interpretation. Studies on dyslexia are approached from
an educational, psychological, and medical aspect and unfortunately there is a wide variation of definitions. The following
terms are sometimes used synonymously with dyslexia: primary
reading disability,[6] specific developmental dyslexia,[7] congenital
word blindness,[8] strephosymbolia,[9] specific reading disability,[10]
developmental lag.[11]

However, the general agreement is that, there is no uniform
etiology for dyslexia. Dyslexia usually refers to those who have
normal intelligence, who have an absence of sensory deficits, an
absence of gross neurological impairment, and who have had
conventional teaching, thought to be necessary for the development of reading. Some authors do not specify that normal intelligence is a necessary requisite, since many children with IQ
below 90 might still have a language disability superimposed
on inadequate capacity to learn.

The estimates of reading failure may be 20%–40% of the school population. This percentage applies to the average school system with perhaps a higher incidence of failure in the inner city school system and a figure down to 5% in the private school system. We do not know if the nationwide patterns of reading achievement are due to selective population effects or if some schools actually do significantly better jobs in the teaching of reading. The attempt to isolate dyslexia as a special entity unrelated to reading disorder will do much to confuse appropriate educational direction. There is no single technique which remediates the problem of dyslexia. The tendency to label all reading problems as dyslexia is erroneous and should be reserved for those children who reading achievement is well below their mental age, who show no evidence of any peripheral sensory defect as blindness or deafness, and show occasional confusion in orientation of letters. Most often there is also a family history of a language disorder.

Many excellent books have been written on a variety of reading difficulties. The bulk of this material, however, deals with the educational process, with teaching methods and corrective and remedial training. Since there is little agreement among many of the writers on any of these subjects, this book is an attempt to clarify the interrelationship of medicine and education. With all that has been written, there is still very little authoritative background available on the basic causes of reading disability. This is true to a great extent because the process of reading is extremely complex. There is a great deal about the problem that is still not understood, for it involves the most intricate mechanism known to man—the human brain.

Reading with understanding is a complicated procedure that involves psychological, physiological, and anatomical factors. Both the learning process and those conditions which may inhibit it will be discussed in greater detail in later chapters. However, most of us can benefit from being reminded of the essentials of this complex process.

Vision only begins the learning process; this retinal stimulus continues, in the form of nerve impulses, along axons through the optic nerve and consecutively to the lateral geniculate body, and then to the occipital lobe of the brain. The impulse proceeds from the occipital lobe through the parietal and temporal lobes to the frontal lobe, where understanding takes place.

Vision involves not only the peripheral aspects of retinal stimulation but also the phenomenon of perception. It is a beginning of the complexities of factors involved in learning. Memory retention and recall are challenged in the learning process. In other words, after perception, memory or retention takes place. When the effectiveness of memory is to be demonstrated, recall occurs. For example, when you glance around a room you may observe the people in the room, at the furnishings, or at objects generally, without any specific attention. You are merely becoming oriented or getting a vague awareness. However, when you concentrate upon one person or one object in the room, there is activation. This is what you will remember, and it will be subject to recall.

The perceptual process enables the student to see the letters D O G which are then mentally transformed into the animate object and an understanding of a real and particular animal. Here, visual perception is reinforced by other stored memories or stimuli—of having heard a barking dog, of having smelled a dog's odor, and of having felt a dog's fur and tail. Through such a complex process, the letters D O G are translated by sensory stimuli into a pluri-dimensional conception and an emotional understanding of what the three letters signify.

At almost any point, this process of reading with understanding can be diminished or blocked by a number of factors. For example, if you teach an animal a learned act and then strike him on the head moderately hard or inject a drug (such as neosynephrine) into his bloodstream, the animal will be unable to learn. This is because certain humoral and biochemical changes take place, during the physiological process of learning and emotions and drugs can alter learning. In a human, fear or anxiety makes adrenalin circulate and, incidentally, inhibit memory. In the brain, cells called astrocytes are concerned with memory and memory effectiveness. During the learning process, the number of such cells that are stimulated determines the amount of concentration and learning that a child is able to exhibit. RNA and DNA are protein materials that reside in these cells. During periods of altered metabolism of the cells, variations of RNA and DNA occur. In the child with cerebral dysfunction some of the astrocytes are damaged or inhibited, or may show some chemical deviation not yet understood.

Children with learning problems can be divided into two major groups.[12] The first consists of those who have what is referred to as *primary* reading retardation. This group includes those children in whom there is obvious brain damage. An example would be a child with cerebral palsy. The group also includes children who seem to have a basic incapacity to integrate or interpret written material and to associate concepts with symbols. Such limitations may be the result of brain injury, of some discrepancy in their development, or of an imbalance in chemical metabolism. Although this segment of the primary reading-retarded group has no observable gross neurological anomaly, there may be subtle neurological changes. There may be problematic motor and sensory changes which can be detected by the more sophisticated psychological examinations. Those children who are classified in the primary retardation group are characterized by resistance to retraining by all techniques used in special education.

The second group, those who have what is termed *secondary* reading retardation, includes children whose reading achievement is poor, but who have normal intelligence and no defects in basic learning capacity. External factors, such as educational problems, environmental factors, and emotional disturbances, are the usual causes of disability in these children. These external factors can be successfully treated by specific teaching methods or with the aid of psychiatric guidance.

The failure of some children to keep up in reading ability with others of their own age has been the subject of a great deal of conjecture. Because so little is known about this condition, a child's inability to interpret written material sucessfully has been blamed upon any number of things. Vision has been accused, with many spokesmen saying that it is because the eye muscles do not function properly. Others assail heredity as the cause. Some say that poor reading is related to lack of cerebral dominance. Still other observers blame diseases of the blood. Even the improper functioning of the thyroid gland and of the other ductless glands have been mentioned as causes of reading retardation. The fact is that none of these assumptions has been adequately substantiated.

Basic to a comprehension of the reading problem is an understanding of the term "reading readiness."[13] Each child who begins school has a varied and different physical, emotional, and educational background. Yet traditionally, at the moment the child reaches six years of age, the parents, the teacher, and society in general expect him to be ready for reading.

Under ideal conditions, the child is prepared to make an easy transition from oral language to written language. He learns to listen, then to talk; he learns how language is organized in the form of sentences and paragraphs. This combination of concepts, attitudes, and interests provides the foundation upon which reading ability is built. It takes 5 to 8 years to develop this reading readiness.[14] With each child there is some variation in the facility he shows for reading readiness. At the strategic age of six years, many factors might influence or retard the coordinated development of his reading skill and play a prominent part in the causation of a reading problem.

In describing the reading problem, a sharp distinction must be made between the "slow" reader and the "retarded" reader. The slow reader is one who reads below his grade level, but whose level of reading is consistent with his intelligence level. On the other hand, a retarded reader is one who reads below his grade level but who may be of higher-than-average intelligence.

For "slow" readers who are intellectually retarded, various plans for education have been developed. Special classes have been set up. Attempts should be made to provide these students with help that will enable them to lead most nearly normal and self-directing lives. The futility of attempting to teach them information and learning processes beyond their capacities has been fairly widely recognized and accepted. Instead of trying to teach material beyond the grasp of these students, teachers should make appropriate adjustments in the educational programs which these children follow.

Unfortunately, unequivocal steps are not yet known in caring for those children who fail in reading, but who are otherwise alert and intelligent. Such a person is an especially tragic figure. He possesses normal mental ability; yet because of factors not completely understood, he finds that he cannot read. There is a delay or a difficulty in learning to read which is out of harmony with his intellectual ability. Too often and for too long this child, who fails *not because of limited intelligence but for other reasons,* has been neglected. In many instances, he has been labeled as a child of low mental capacity and therefore has not been expected to achieve. Equally tragic is the fact that he has usually been placed with children of limited intelligence, and provided with the same type of educational program as that designed for a retarded child or slow learner.

In other cases, the dyslexic reader has been considered lazy and unwilling to learn. Parents and teachers alike may have recognized that he is not unintelligent. He will speak and act intelligently about things that interest him. He does well in out-of-school activities which obviously require an alert, intelligent mind. So, parents and teachers reach the conclusion that the only explanation can be that he does not *try* to do well in school. They become convinced that a bit of determined effort is all it will take for him to achieve. For such reasons, a child of this type frequently has not been promoted in school, particularly as punishment for his "laziness," but also in an honest effort to shock him into putting forth the effort to learn. In addition, he has been goaded and threatened at home, kept in at night to do extra work, drilled on work assigned for the next day. The main result has nearly always been the total frustration of both parent and child.

The most typical characteristics of a student with a dyslexic problem can be described as follows:

He is usually a male student of normal or superior intelligence.[15] He may be left-handed or ambidextrous. There is a persistence of a normal childhood tendency to reverse letters and symbols, such as p for q, or u for n. There is also a tendency to reverse words, such as *stop* for *pots,* and *was* for *saw.* He may show a tendency to read from right to left. In rare cases there is actual "mirror writing," a reverse writing intelligible only when viewed in a mirror.

The child may be unable to work out the pronunciation of a strange word. He may fail to see similarities and differences in forms, or in words such as *on* and *no,* or *pub* and *bud.* He may not hear differences in sounds of letters; or in reading he may be unable to keep his place in sentences. He may vocalize the words and still be unable to read with sufficient understanding. The child may later present an emotional problem, reading two or three grades below his own grade level, but often doing better than average in arithmetic.

Workers in the field of special education have pointed out many causes for the inability to read well, but efforts to correct the condition are not uniformally successful. Corrective treatment usually is not provided until the deficiency in reading is demonstrated by repeated failure. Unless something effective is done to cope with this growing problem, the need for remedial reading classes and clinics will soon reach such proportions that training classes for children with learning disabilities will form a separate and substantial subdivision of all departments of education. Current estimates say that there are as many as 24 million functional illiterates in the United States.

Special reading instruction, furthermore, is often subject to the advocacy of faddists who offer many types of therapy, with little thought given to the primary causes of the reading disturbance. It is not only teachers, but reading clinicians as well, who often use terms such as "emotional block," "anxious parents," and "brain damage" to dismiss a problem that they do not understand.

Research has emphasized the complexities of the problem rather than the solutions. Since there are few controlled studies for remediation, educators and others have turned to panaceas and pseudoscientific methods which are usually justified by articles that appear in popular magazines rather than in professional journals which should be critical of their content. Instead of expounding methods of treatment based on the enthusiasm of vested interests, we should adopt as guidelines for education controlled basic research which is unbiased and applicable to large groups of students rather than a select few.

Because of the complexity that reading difficulties have demonstrated, there is a growing insistence that educators, physicians, and other professionals should work together closely to find the elusive answers to the reading retardation problem.

In the past few years, the author has seen four children of ages five through eight who were far advanced in their ability to read. It was recorded that these children read as early as three years of age. They were quite compulsive in their reading and were able to read fifth grade to seventh grade materials. Not only could they read English but they were adept in reading other languages. Their IQ's were within normal range. From their histories, it was noted that they would make a habit, early in life, of reading posters and television commercial advertisements. They had taught themselves by phonetic ability to read far beyond their intellectual capacity. Other cases of this type have been reported. This type of case has been identified as hyperlexia.

The incursion of medicine into education has been brought about because there is a growing consensus of opinion that a substantial number of cases of reading failure do not result simply from poor teaching, lack of social and cultural opportunities, or motivational lack, but are perhaps aggravated by specific defects in the central nervous system that cause perceptual difficulties. These children *cannot* unscramble symbols which reach the brain by the auditory or visual pathways.[16]

The purpose of this book is to provide an understanding of both the educational and medical aspects of reading and show how they are interrelated in reading disabilities. The following chapters are intended to present comprehensive information for parents, educators, psychologists and physicians, all of whom are inevitably involved with the reading problem.

Early Predictive Studies

Predictive studies should better provide the answer to why some children progress slowly and require many years of special education before returning to regular classes, and even why some children are never able to return to regular classroom situations.

Which children benefit the most from special education and by which methods of treatment can they best be helped? Uniform methods of teaching are not applicable to all children, and a "paint spray" approach is only going to lead to programs that are not identified. Interpretations of the results obtained in such programs will have little validity for the global education of children removed from the community in which the research is performed. The greatest strength of early predictive diagnosis is that it leads to a preventive approach seeking to avoid or minimize learning disabilities before their development.

Ideally, a child with a real or potential learning difficulty should be identified before beginning school or, certainly, by first grade. If this could be accomplished, a teacher would be able to outline for the child an academic program that could be adjusted to the ways in which he would be enabled to learn and perhaps to suggest the pace at which learning should proceed. The growing number of children with reading disabilities makes it imperative that there should be some way to differentiate the intellectual capacities of these children and adjust their goals so that they can be made to coincide more realistically with their aptitudes. One of our most important contributions in dealing with the problem of reading disabilities may well be made in the area of early predictive studies.

Psychologists and educators have always sought a measure which would sort out and differentiate the capabilities of school pupils. Millions of children take IQ tests every year, but these tests are under heavy criticism. Some critics say that the tests are culturally biased and even that the component tests do not add up to a measure of intelligence at all.

The first tests of mental measurement were designed by Sir Francis Galton, who tried to prove that intelligence was inherited. In 1905 the French psychologist, Alfred Binet, developed a series of tests to identify mentally defective children. From the administration of his tests to large numbers of children of various ages, he derived the concept of "mental age." Lewis M. Terman, an American psychologist, later developed the concept of "intelligence quotient." By dividing the mental age of a child by his chronological age, and multiplying the result by 100, one could obtain the IQ (intelligence quotient) score of the child. Terman revised the Binet test so as to identify the most capable children, in order that they could have educational and cultural advantages that would prepare them for leadership. This revision was known as the Stanford-Binet Test.

It must be remembered that an intelligence test is meaningful only under carefully controlled conditions of individual testing, preferably by a trained psychologist, who can bring out the best of a child's ability to perform and who can remain sensitive to the level of the child's motivation during the testing situation.

An IQ score, furthermore, is not a fixed score. Fluctuations can occur because of physical, emotional, and cultural changes. One group of children, for example, contained some who, after psychotherapy, increased their IQ scores by as much as 40 points. It has also been found that children from homes which provided them poor cultural stimulation did poorly on the IQ tests. Groups of such children who were taken to libraries, zoos, and museums, showed an increase in IQ.

John P. Ertl and Dr. William Barry[17] recently used the visually evoked response (VER) as a method of measuring intelligence. The VER is done by exposing the child to tachistoscopic stimuli while electrodes placed on the head record the electrical sensations received in the brain. These individual recordings are computerized, summated, and averaged and the final VER wave is produced. They tested the underlying neurologic efficiency on which intelligence depends. Connors[18] has described a family of poor readers who had a change in electroencephalographic (EEG) wave form of the visually evoked response in the left parietal area of the brain. Studies of two samples of poor readers, and a sample of children with contrasting verbal-performance discrepancies on the Weschler Intelligence Scale for Children (WISC), showed significant relationships between verbal skills and the late components of the VER. The strongest VER amplitude correlations occur in the left parietal area. Children with verbal-performance discrepancies on the WISC also showed highly significant latency effects in the late waves of the VER.

Amplitude changes of wave forms in the left parietal area suggest an alteration in the information processing capabilities of this area in reading disorders. Test data indicate that children with low performance IQs are more impaired neurologically and thus would have poorer results on the performance part of the WISC.[19]

Although it is too early to be certain, it is hoped that the VER might be an instrument that could be used in early identification of the child with learning disability. Subsequent investigations should provide more information as to the reliability of the VER and its role in the investigation of learning disabilities.

Since, in the past, there were no predictive studies except that of teacher estimate that could be used in the kindergarten or first-grade level, many children, some immature and some intellectually unequal to the tasks of first grade, were placed in a learning situation with which they could not cope. These children were not intellectually prepared to compete with their peers in the normal classroom situation.

A very significant report by Schiffman[20] indicates that if the potential learning disability in children was diagnosed in the second grade, 82% of them could be brought back to grade level in a two-year period by appropriate teaching methods. However, if the learning-disabled child was not identified until after the fourth grade, it was found that only 15% could be readily remediated. The others, despite the use of sophisticated methods, became chronic failures.

Schiffman's work included the success and failure rate of children at all levels; the following Table shows the results of his investigation:

Table I
Schiffman's Results

Learning Disability Diagnosed in	Successful Remediation
Grade 2	82%
Grade 3	46%
Grade 4	42%
Grade 5	15%
Grade 6	8%
Grade 7	10%
Grade 8	11%
Grade 9	6%

This Table is based on a review of 10,000 cases; the rate of successful remedial treatment depends upon the grade at which the child is identified as having a learning disability. This is a very significant contribution and emphasizes the advantages and the need for the early diagnosis of learning difficulty.

Consideration of factors in identification should begin at birth. Features identifiable at this period and correlated with intelligence were suggested by Hardy[21] when investigating children whom she studied in the Johns Hopkins Collaborative Project. High Apgar scores, elevated bilirubin blood levels, and a birth weight below 1500 grams have all been correlated to minimal brain dysfunction, lower intelligence, and reading failure.

Other correlations were attempted by Castner in 1935.[22] From his studies, Castner identified certain characteristics of the child and related these to the probable progress of the child. Unfortunately, his work was soon forgotten. Not until 1959 was a significant resumption of a similar effort made. In 1968

DeHirsch[23] published an excellent book on early predictive studies, in which she attempted to identify children who might have difficulties in the school system. The purpose of this study was not only to predict success or failure, but to offer suggestions on how to protect the child who might be a high-risk student in the normal learning situation. By protecting such a child, and perhaps by utilizing different techniques of teaching, it was suggested that this high-risk child could become a successful reader and experience success devoid of frustration. These studies of DeHirsch and Jansky will be reported in detail because their studies are the most valid among predictability studies.

Among the well-known achievement tests are the Stanford Achievement, Iowa Tests of Education Development, and the Metropolitan Tests. A visual-motor Gestalt test by Lauretta Bender is easy to use and provides much information on many levels. It can be obtained from the American Orthopsychiatric Association (Monograph #3, 1938). The Frostig Tests identify and train in five areas of visual-motor perception. The Gates-MacGinitie Testing Program in Reading is designed for groups and gives measures of individual silent-reading skill. The Goodenough Measurements of Intelligence by drawings published by the World Book Company in 1926 is of value as a projective test; it has been revised by Dale Harris and published by Harcourt, Brace & World, 1963. For further references in the area of the nature, recognition, and treatment of language difficulties, the reader is referred to an excellent bibliography by Margaret B. Rawson,[24] published by the Orton Society, 1971.

Readiness tests which have importance in the identification of children with learning disabilities are:

1. Lee Clark
2. PMA
3. Gates MacGinitie
4. Slingerland
5. Meeting Street School Screening Test (MSSST)
6. Metropolitan
7. DeHirsch & Jansky
8. Wechsler Intelligence Test for Children (WISC)

The Slingerland Screening Tests[25] have had widespread use as a screening program. There are no standardized national norms, since the authors prefer that each community develop its own standards with relevance to the child's particular social and educational exposure. Based on these factors there will be marked differences among the children from school to school in both kind and level of performance.

Slingerland has noted that one set of norms would not be applicable to all groups of children and each group must be developed to cover children from various cultures and a varying socioeconomic status. However, there is a strong assumption that her local standards would also apply nationally.

DeHirsch and Jansky's contributions remain the most significant in the field of early predictive studies. The pilot study of the feasibility of early prediction directed by Katrina DeHirsch, with Jeannette Jansky and William S. Lankford as co-investigators[26] sought to determine which of 50 or so children at the kindergarten level were likely to fail in reading two years later. First, they presented 37 variables to these kindergarten children. The product of these 37 tests was a 10-test battery called the Predictive Index. This Index was the result of those tests given in kindergarten that had the highest coefficient of correlation with second-grade reading, and also those that best separated the failing readers from the remainder of the group. The 10 tests found to make up this Predictive Index were: (1) Pencil Use, (2) Bender Motor Gestalt, (3) Wepman Auditory Discrimination, (4) Categories, (5) Number of Words Used in Telling a Story, (6) the Word Matching subtest of the Gates Reading Readiness Battery, (7) the Horst Matching Test, (8) two Word Learning tests, (9) a Spelling Learning task, and (10) Letter Naming tests.

Of the original group of kindergarten children, these 10 tests had identified 10 of the 11 children who subsequently failed reading at the end of Grade 2. Upon completion of this study, it was evident that an effort would have to be made to validate these tests: i.e., to give them to a much larger sampling of children in order to determine their general usefulness and reliability as early predictors. This research was carried out by Jeannette Jansky[27] in undertaking the second phase of the early prediction research.

They were moved by the commitment to test, in a fairly rigorous fashion, the 10 test Predictive Index developed in the first study. They were also influenced to investigate leads relative to changes in the understanding of the problems of prediction. By the time the research plan for the second study was being formulated, a number of people had already started to use the Predictive Index. They were seeking a shorter instrument, which could easily be administered by school personnel or aides to large groups of five-year-olds. It was desirable to devise such a battery; also, there was much interest in trying several measures not included among the 37 kindergarten tests originally administered to children in the first study. Thus, while it was planned to validate the Predictive Index on a second group of children, the major concern of Phase 2 shifted to the preparation of a shorter instrument which would probably be useful to more people.

The subjects for the second study were kindergarten children drawn from five public schools in two districts of New York City. The kindergarten tests were administered to all children who spoke and understood conversational English. Of the group of 508 children tested as kindergarteners, 341 continued to attend the schools in which they had originally been enrolled and were available for evaluation two years later. Sixty more of the original group were located, so that the final sample consisted of 401 subjects to whom both kindergarten and second-grade tests had been administered.

About 50% of the children were white, 42% were black, while the remaining were Puerto Rican, with a very few Chinese children. The white children were, on the average, significantly less disadvantaged than were the blacks and Puerto Ricans. As second graders, the children tended to receive at least average scores on the WISC. However, the range in scores on the subtests was quite wide.

The kindergarten tests were administered individually to the children at their schools in the spring of the kindergarten year. Additional tests were included to increase the number of measures in certain categories. These were: Letter Naming Test, Number of Words Used in Telling a Story, the Minnesota Perceptual Diagnostic Test (which involved the copying of designs and calculating the extent to which they were rotated), Sentence Memory items from the 1937 Stanford-Binet, a Picture Naming task, the Roswell-Chall Auditory Blending Test, a clinical assessment of Oral Language Level, and a measure of the child's tendency to Use Configuration for Word Matching.

The first problem of the second phase of this research was to see how the Predictive Index from the first study would work with the new group of children. The evaluation of the Predictive Index was based on its performance when used with three new groups of children. Some conclusions drawn from the findings in the second testing and relating to validation of the Predictive Index developed in the first study may be summarized as follows: The old Predictive Index varied in efficiency when used with new samples. The accuracy with which the failing readers were identified varied from sample to sample. Because of population differences, norms changed within the individual school and norms developed for one population do not hold for another. The Predictive Index as used with the heterogeneous group of 300 kindergarten children was most efficient in preselecting the best of the second-grade readers. The Predictive Index also seemed to function most efficiently in identifying the failing readers when used with children whose IQ clustered around 100. When administered to the subgroup of 50 children matched to first-study subjects, the Index's performance was satisfactory and the results were nearly identical to those of the earlier research.

The major goal of the second study was to devise a screening test that could be administered quickly and that would, therefore, be useful for large, heterogeneous populations. As with the first study, a cutoff point was selected which resulted in catching as many actual reading failures and introducing as few false positives (children who later passed) as possible.

In Jansky's second efforts, a group of five tests was selected as predictors. The battery developed included the Letter Naming, Picture Naming tests, the Gates Word Matching, the Bender, and the Sentence Memory tests as additional contributors. This short screening battery correctly identified 79% of the failing readers. It picked up only 22% of the children who actually passed.

It should be pointed out that to achieve high accuracy rates in individual prediction it is essential to take advantage of the kindergarten teacher's knowledge of her children. In the process of formulating clinical predictions, the teacher sifts and weighs *all* she knows about a child to arrive at her prognostication of how he will perform later on. Although teachers' predictions alone are not sufficient, they do represent a valuable source of information to be checked against so-called "hard" data. There is no need to view clinical and statistical prediction as mutually exclusive.

The need for research in early identification is recognized by others. Prominent among these is a series of tests known as the Meeting Street School Screening Test (MSSST).[28] This test seeks to identify kindergarten and first-grade children who do not possess language and visual-or-auditory-perceptual skills to process adequately the symbolic information required in the school curriculum. It is recognized that if young children with potential difficulties could be reliably identified, it might be possible to reduce the large number of children who later manifest learning disabilities and emotional reactions.

There is one final point. It is best to test kindergarten children individually. If the battery is short enough—and if the screening batteries take only 15 minutes to administer—individual testing is feasible. Group testing simply adds to the existing difficulty of getting a representative sample of a five-year-old's performance. Observation of hundreds of five-year-olds suggests that they are not particularly test-wise; many cannot give a good indication of what they know if left by themselves to work on a group test using paper and pencil. A number of them who will become fine readers are still preoccupied or distracted by the effort required for grapho-motor expression. The time taken to test them singly is well worth it.

In summary, there is a clear need for individualizing prediction. Accurate prediction is certainly possible and the methodology is available. We still must use caution in any testing situation. But with what we already know about the child and the objective measures of his relative performance on tests, it is relevant to conclude that tests are available which are closely related to reading success. Prediction involves collecting the relevant information about the child and considering it systematically, but prediction can be accurate only to the degree that it is highly individual.

It is certainly true that if a child has an IQ of 120 and his observed behavior is equivalent to that of other children with comparable intelligence, we can reasonably expect the child to perform normally in academic pursuits. However, there is an excellent equation that deals with this expectancy and it may be put down as $E \neq O = T$. Translated, this means: If "expectancy" of the child is not correlated with the "observable behavior," then "trouble" can be expected. Thus, if a child's IQ is 60, and this is not correlated realistically with the future goals of the child, then that child is headed for trouble.

The purpose of predictive tests at the preschool or first-grade level should be not only to differentiate children of varying learning capacities, but to attempt to identify the specific area of handicap so that a program can be outlined to enable the children to work around their areas of deficiency. This is related to the work being done by Mark[29] which involves an effort to identify a specific deficit so that failure can be averted. The prospects of remedial success are vastly brighter if a child's learning disability can be recognized before he becomes enmeshed in a pattern of frustration and failure. One of the purposes of this book is to encourage the identification of the different causes of a learning disability—such as the visual, auditory, neurological, or educational factors. Equally important is the attempt to present persuasive evidence that one should not attempt to teach *to* a child's area of deficiency, but to teach around it, so that through his other, unimpaired capabilities, the child's learning efforts may be enhanced and his educational goals achieved with greater ease.

Psychological Evaluation

The psychological evaluation of a child with a reading disability is an important part of the effort to rehabilitate the child. Because of the possibility of many etiological factors which may be significant, the child should be referred for a profile examination. The psychological evaluation is extremely important as a means of identifying the child's intellectual capacity (or IQ). Such an evaluation will assist in identifying the child as either a developmental, a corrective, or a remedial reader.

A developmental reader is a child who works within the limits of his basic intellectual capacity. If his IQ is 120 and he performs at a level commensurate with his ability, then this child is successfully doing what he is capable of doing. If the child's IQ is 70 and he performs at that level, then he too is achieving commensurate with intellectual capacity. The developmental reader, then, is one who is applying reading skills in a systematic way commensurate with his potential. Approximately 60% of the children in our schools are developmental readers.

The second group of children whom we seek to identify are the corrective readers, a group who read below grade level even though possessing normal intelligence. This group falls into Rabinovitch's classification, which he calls a "secondary" type.

The cause of reading failure among children in this group is not lowered intelligence but is due to other exogenous factors such as a psychiatric, an educational, or perhaps a physical disability which impedes learning. This group contains approximately 25% of the reading-disabled population. In a normal classroom situation, they can usually be brought to grade level with the proper corrective methods.

In the third group, one finds the remedial reader. This is a student with normal or high intelligence, characterized by persistent failure in spite of normal classroom teaching efforts. He is the child who frequently reverses his letters and words. He confuses *d* with *b* or reads *saw* for *was*. Often there is some degree of difficulty in laterality or dominance, and, above all, his deficiency is marked, for he reads two or more grades below grade level. Two to ten percent of school children fall into this group of remedial readers, popularly identified as dyslexic children. This classification is important when evaluations of remedial programs are to be considered. Methods of therapy applicable to one group cannot be claimed as being applicable to other groups.

There are other advantages of the psychological evaluation, since it does provide an evaluation of the emotional attitudes of the child. In addition, the psychological profile hopefully will reveal those channels of teaching that can be effectively used for the instruction of the reading-disabled child.

In other words, some of the probable factors which have been responsible for, or may be contributing to, the child's failure need to be determined and a way formulated by which an individual program of remediation can be successful.

If a reading disability exists it is important to isolate this disability; the student should not be penalized in subjects which are dependent on reading, such as history, social studies, and geography. He should be provided with special learning opportunities (using other than written materials) so he can learn the informational content consistent with grade-level subjects. This might involve the use of records, films, and tapes. A specific learning disability program should afford the best setting for this type of requirement. An effort should be made to keep the child with his age group (social peers), so that he will be with children who share his basic social and intellectual interests. This is a form of "circumvention."

A phenomenon worthy of mention is the "balloon effect." This effect is most often applicable to the student in grades 7–12. It involves a child with a reading disability who is just managing to keep on grade level with most subjects, but who always fails one of the group of subjects. If special attention is paid to that one failing subject, it can be brought to grade level. But then he fails in another subject. The reason is that he cannot, because of his reading disability, handle too many subjects. It would be better if a limited schedule were pursued so that success could be achieved in all subjects.

Therefore it is necessary to identify parameters which may have an effect upon the reading ability of the child. It is well-known that intelligence is positively related to reading ability. In most cases, if the child's intelligence is average or above, he should have sufficient cognitive potential for the development of adequate reading skills. Therefore, if in the process of the psychological evaluation of a disabled reader it is found that the child has an intellectual capacity which is average or above, one should suspect that there are other factors which are interfering with the child's reading achievement.

There are, of course, many factors which may interfere with the achievement of maximum score on an intelligence test, so that the IQ obtained may not always truly represent the child's intelligence. Some of these factors that interfere with intelligence testing might be special sensory defects, neuro-muscular diseases, emotional disorders, and cultural deprivation. Furthermore, the child may possess some cognitive skills which are not adequately revealed by the intelligence test.

The psychological examination in the reading-age child is preferably measured by the Wechsler Intelligence Scale for Children, known familiarly as the WISC.[30] Three separate IQ scores are yielded by the WISC: a Verbal IQ, a Performance IQ, and a Full-Scale I.Q. score, which is derived from the performance and verbal scores. The WISC is normally reported by the Full-Scale score. Actually, this does not tell the entire story about a child's abilities. There might be a large discrepancy between the Verbal and Performance subtests or there may be a deficiency in one or another of the subtests of the verbal or the performance areas, which could materially affect the total Verbal or Performance tests. As frequently happens, the child may receive a Full-Scale IQ score of 80 only because he was deficient in one or two of the various subtests which make up the WISC.

The verbal and the performance parts of the WISC are each based upon a series of eleven standardized subtests. The Verbal score contains 6 subtests involving (1) information, (2) comprehension, (3) arithmetic, (4) similarities, (5) vocabulary, and (6) digit span tests. This group is frequently called the auditory part of the WISC. The performance part of the WISC is often concerned with the visual factors. These 5 subtests consist of (1) picture completion, (2) picture arrangement, (3) block design, (4) object assembly, and (5) coding.

The verbal subtests as a group are directed toward an assessment of the child's ability to understand and use language, while the performance subtests are directed toward an assessment of visual-perceptive skills, but almost all of these tests are verbally weighted, as in the Block Design subtest, where the child is required to duplicate a printed design with blocks. By inspection of the subtest scaled scores which are usually included in the psychological report, one may determine specific strengths and weaknesses of the child. Normally, the Verbal IQ and Performance IQ are within 5 to 10 points of each other. Excessive discrepancies may be of diagnostic significance. Thus a low score on the performance subtests could not only indicate a perceptual-motor impairment, but could also support the influence of emotional factors which could inhibit the child's concentration during reading and other intellectual tasks. A high score on the subtests might suggest strengths which could be capitalized upon in a remedial reading program.

Despite adequate intelligence, personality traits and emotional attitudes often interfere with the development of adequate reading skills. The child who is rebellious, negativistic, and hostile toward authority is quite different from one who is excessively immature, dependent, and emotionally withdrawn. Yet the behavior of each may, in an academic setting, effectively prevent the child from learning to read and generally interfere with school progress.

To assess the psychodynamics of personality integration, projective personality tests such as the Rorschach Psychodiagnostic Test, the Thematic Apperception Test (TAT), or the

Children's Apperception Test (CAT) are frequently administered.[31]

The Rorschach Psychodiagnostic Test is a series of 10 ink-blot cards. The subject is shown each card and asked to respond verbally as to its content. Since the subject matter of the blots is ambiguous, the individual must project his own thoughts into the picture in order to arrive at a meaningful interpretation. Scoring on norms gives the probability of response which might allow the examiner to evaluate the emotional status of the subject.

The TAT and the CAT are less ambiguous than the Rorschach Test in that structured pictures are presented to the subject. Most TAT cards present human figures in poses suggesting high emotional content, while the CAT cards present animals in various poses. In each case the subject is asked to tell a brief story about the picture. The content or theme of the story allows the examiner to obtain insight regarding the emotional relationships between the subject and significant persons in his psychosocial environment.

These projective tests may be complemented by psycho-motor tests such as the Bender Visual-Motor Gestalt Test or the Draw-a-Person Test. The Bender Visual-Motor Gestalt Test[32] is a series of nine geometric figures each presented on individual cards which the subject is asked to duplicate. Gross deficiencies in the reproduction of the Bender designs may indicate central nervous system dysfunction, marked psychopathology, or simply developmental immaturity. Quite frequently it is difficult, if not impossible, to determine which of these three factors is primarily responsible for an abnormal record.

In the Draw-a-Person Test[33] the subject is presented with a blank sheet of paper and requested to "draw a person." Neither the sex nor the age is specified. After the subject draws the first picture he is then asked to draw the opposite sex. The quality of the drawings may be scored against age norms, and the percentile rank of the individual may be suggestive of advanced, normal, or retarded psychomaturational level. The test is not, of course, to be considered in isolation, but in the context of the total test battery. While standardized administration of psychological tests is usually desirable, examinations administered under stress, such as, for example, that brought on by the presence of a parent, are often of diagnostic significance in elucidating parent-child psychopathology. Intelligence and personality testing is complemented by clinical interviewing, which yields in the hands of a skilled clinician information equally important to that obtained by the clinical tests. It is desirable to individually interview the patient, each parent, and if possible, one or more of the school personnel most familiar with the child's educational progress. Independent interviews with each parent are particularly valuable since one often obtains widely divergent narratives regarding the child's reading disability.

The diagnostic reading evaluation may be included as an aspect of the psychological evaluation, or it may be administered separately by a diagnostic reading specialist. In either case it should be performed by a clinician experienced in educational diagnosis, using one of the more widely accepted reading-analysis tests, such as the Durrell Analysis of Reading Difficulty or the Gates-McKillop Reading Tests. A thorough reading analysis will provide separate grade-equivalent scores for rate, accuracy, and comprehension in both oral and silent reading, and usually some indication of the child's learning ability. The analysis will also include grade-equivalency scores for listening comprehension, sight vocabulary, visual memory of word forms, phonic analysis of word elements, and knowledge of auditory blending, handwriting, and spelling. In addition to the reading analysis, it is important to test the child's achievement in other subjects, especially arithmetic, for comparison with reading level. In some cases, the child is equally retarded in reading and mathematics, while in other cases the child's disability may be limited primarily to reading. In addition to the objective reading tests, the child's behavioral and emotional reactions while reading may be of significant diagnostic importance. Some children are so anxious while attempting to read that they are unable to utilize the skills they may have, while others may escape the frustrations of failure by negativism or acting-out behavior.

There have been those who claimed that if a child scored high in performance and low in verbal ability on the WISC, the child has dyslexia. Or there is the claim that the reverse is true, that dyslexia is present if the child has a high verbal score and a low score on performance. Actually, it does not matter which of these scores is higher—the verbal or the performance. The important thing is to know how to analyze a WISC score through a study of its full range of subtests.

For example, one should look at all of the subtest scores to see if perhaps there is an area of marked deficiency. It is possible that a child may be extremely deficient in digit span. If this is the case, it would suggest the child can hear but he has poor short-term memory, and it is in the processing of verbal instructions that the child might have his difficulty. In such a case, we might simply select optimal treatment and the best teaching strategy to circumvent that area of the child's deficiency.

There are many children who may have some specific defect, in which the score on one of the performance subtests is minimized, thus lowering the entire performance score. Therefore, anyone who is to interpret the WISC test should have access to scores on all of the individual subtests of the WISC, so that a proper treatment design can be formulated for the child's future education. The cause of the child's difficulty may not be and need not be brain dysfunction, nor need it be the fact that he has a low IQ, because he may show low ability in some areas but remarkably high ability in others. Thus a general, overall study of scores on the various parts of the WISC will enable one to isolate those factors which cause deficiencies. Learning does not progress evenly and this results in areas or patterns of intellectual strength and weakness.

Standard psychometric tests such as the Cattell, Griffith, Binet, WISC, WAIS, Grace Arthur, Eisenson, Bender, and Benton make up the bulk of the testing procedures. Henry Mark has developed tests consisting of items from all of these tests. This enables the examiner to select an optimal testing path, which will generate patient profiles of intellectual capabilities.

The work of Mark is related to this difficulty of psychodiagnostic efforts to isolate specific areas of deficit. In his recent article, "Some Requirements for Translating Psychological Diagnoses into Teaching Programs,"[34] Mark stresses the importance of obtaining useful psychodiagnostic reports on each child. He makes a very strong case for the identification and isolation of that channel of communication in which there might be a deficiency. As is well known, minimal brain dysfunction may differentially affect a child's cognitive skills within specific modalities and languages.

Any child who is having difficulty in school must be given a careful psychological examination directed at identifying his areas of strength and weakness. A good psychological report must contain concepts which will demonstrate that the search for key disorders was done in a comprehensive and systematic fashion, so that there is little likelihood of false positive or negative findings. This concept of searching through test channels to find both specific cognitive skills and specific areas of dysfunction is extremely important if one is to know how to systematize a treatment strategy for the child's improvement.

The teacher who does not understand about the connections and learning channels may commit many major errors in dealing with a child with a learning disability. For example, the teacher is likely to spend excessive time, even years, trying to develop a totally nonfunctioning auditory system. In the same child, she is also apt to spend an inordinate amount of time attempting to develop a kinesthetic system beyond the potential usefulness of that system. In pursuing these two aims in the child, the teacher runs a high risk of not fully utilizing other, more adequate channels of learning. If the child is functionally deaf, the auditory languages may not be fully utilized. By persisting in working with the impossible learning areas, the teacher is likely to invoke in the child serious psychiatric influences, overtones, or background because of the constant frustration and failures which have been imposed upon the child.

A good analogy to what has been said regarding the test channels would be that of a malfunctioning television set. If the television does not function properly, then electronic equipment can differentiate between the input and output systems to determine which "side" of the mechanism has a faulty part. The diagnostic examination of a child suspected of a learning disability should take place in an analogous way. Testing can reveal whether the disability is of peripheral or of central origin, and a complete psychological report can indicate which specific central factor is involved in the learning problem. If properly organized and carried out, this diagnostic examination should take little more time than the diagnosis of a piece of malfunctioning electronic equipment.

Mark has devised a chart in which there is a hierarchy of central nervous system functions of "systems" which emerge in normal development as an ordered set in each of the channels of communication. The emergence order of these systems is compatible with the norms for developmental milestones published by Cattell in 1940,[35] Gesell in 1954,[36] and by Terman and Merrill[37] in 1960. They differ primarily from developmental milestones in that Mark subdivides the systems within each channel into subsystems, subsubsystems, and so on, thereby permitting a more finely grained analysis of a child's learning strengths and weaknesses. Entering mental measurements on a subject into such a chart permits the tester to report systematically not only strengths and weaknesses, but also pseudostrengths ("halo effects") and pseudoweaknesses which often obscure the real mental-ability profile of the person. Furthermore, Mark's diagnostic search strategy is aimed at finding the most basic learning disability which can "account for" the largest number of secondary disabilities within the hierarchy of developmental milestones in each channel. These basic disabilities then automatically become the target of educational treatment and/or circumvention strategies.

After a proper evaluation there will be no wasted time and effort that only brings havoc into the emotional well-being of the child and his family. Rather, by examination of these individual areas of learning skills one can acquire an adequate learning-disability profile. From this profile, a proper teaching technique and strategy might be developed for the individual student.

The psychological evaluation therefore provides a means of indicating which children should be identified as either developmental readers, corrective readers, or remedial readers. With regard to the latter two groups, the analysis should give an indication of the best steps to take toward correction or remediation of the problem. For the dyslexic reader, the psychological evaluation should result in specific recommendations regarding changes in the psychoeducational environment of the individual child which might enable him to achieve adequate reading skills. The range of possible psychoeducational modifications is quite broad, and the specific changes recommended will depend upon the nature of each child's learning disability.

Central Nervous System Dysfunction

In many instances the very medical advances that have saved the lives of children have also increased the number of children with physical disabilities. The phenomenon of brain damage in children offers a striking example of this process. Many children who, before the era of antibiotic treatment and other lifesaving techniques, would have died at birth, or from such diseases as meningitis or encephalitis, today survive—but they bear the marks of these ordeals in the form of so-called "brain damage."

For those children with brain damage that produces cerebral palsy, epilepsy, or mental retardation, both research and service are becoming increasingly available. But there are many children whose brain damage is less readily detected and whose manifestations are perceptual rather than motor. These children are largely unprovided for in the present educational system. They are frequently misunderstood and labeled "problem children" by their perplexed parents and teachers, who often find them intractable and resistant to proper education.

The case of the child whose reading problem results from brain damage is possibly the most perplexing of all cases of reading retardation, for his is the most difficult to diagnose. Even if he has minimal brain damage or cerebral dysfunction, the child may appear to be completely normal. A physical examination will frequently show nothing abnormal, and his intelligence may be normal, or even above normal. A sizable number of children of normal or superior intelligence have reading difficulties because they suffer some degree of brain dysfunction which does not reveal itself in any obvious manner.

It is important that physicians and teachers recognize the symptoms of such dysfunction in handicapped readers. In some cases, the effects of such damage may not evidence itself except in the child's inability to interpret written material or to associate concepts with symbols. On the other hand, researchers have carefully studied children with brain damage and found a number of behavior patterns which are characteristic of this condition. Some of these cases are reviewed here so that behavior of children with brain damage can be better understood.

From 1915 to 1921 a pandemic of encephalitis—sleeping sickness—swept the world. The after-effects of the disease, which causes swelling in the brain, drew a great deal of attention. These cases have been described lucidly by Dr. Frank R. Ford, a Johns Hopkins neurologist[38]:

> There is in most cases no marked reduction of intelligence, but personality changes of a profound nature frequently result. In most cases, physical signs are absent or trivial. These children are very destructive and impulsive. Any impulse which occurs to them is at once translated into action. Their misdeeds are not planned, but are the result of the temptation of the moment. The natural inhibitions of fear of consequence, which restrain all of us from injudicious behavior, seem to be lacking in these children. Without any thought of punishment, they will steal, lie, destroy property, set fires and commit various offenses. They usually make no effort to evade detection, and when reproached with their conduct, will reply that they could not help it. They may be quite indifferent to punishment, or may exhibit exaggerated remorse for their offense, which, however, does not prevent further misdeeds. An important factor in these behavior disorders is the emotional instability. The child's

mood changes in response to the slightest stimulus. Most patients are very restless and overactive, hurrying from one form of mischief to another throughout the day. The children often run away from home and are impatient of any restraint.

There have been occasional reports, one as early as 1892, of the postmortem examination of the brain of a person who had suffered from *alexia*. (*Alexia* is a condition wherein a person has lost his previous ability to recognize letters or words, read and yet is still able to write spontaneously. Alexia is similar to the word *dyslexia*, but dyslexia is usually reserved to describe those who have "word blindness" from birth.) In 1892[39] Dejerine published the first case of a patient who, after having had a cerebrovascular accident (stroke) developed an inability to read. He identified this inability as alexia. A number of years later, this patient died of a major stroke. The postmortem examination of his brain revealed a lesion in the subcortical region of the left angular gyrus, suggesting that a lesion in the left angular gyrus might account for inability to read.

Similarly, children who have brain damage may demonstrate neurological signs that are referable to the parietal lobes. Such lesions in the parietal lobes of the dominant and nondominant hemispheres can each reveal findings that are compatible with signs frequently found in dyslexia.

Lesions in the dominant parietal lobe are suggested by dysgraphia, dyscalculia, finger agnosia, errors in right-left discrimination, dyspraxia, and even dyslexia. Dysfunction in the nondominent parietal lobe is suggested by disorder of body image, unilateral spatial imperception, spatial agnosia, and constructional apraxia.

There are overt signs of damage or injury that a careful neurological examination can on occasion reveal to the pediatric neurologist. But most frequently there are no obvious signs of damage, and this leads to the application of the term "cerebral dysfunction." Either the signs are too minimal or there may only be a dysfunction.

In summary, the following characteristics are present: first, the intelligence as formally measured is normal or only moderately reduced. The full-scale IQ is generally within normal limits, although more careful scrutiny at once brings out some significant points. It is usually low for the expected average for the family, and the scatter within it is remarkably wide. Tests involving rote memory are generally best performed, while those involving step-by-step reasoning from premise to premise, and those involving perception of spatial and form relationships, are done very poorly. The scatter may indeed be so wide that the full-scale IQ becomes quite meaningless. Second, physical signs of neurological abnormality are absent or trivial. Minor inequalities of reflexes, slight asymmetries of growth, occasional strabismus, an occasional extensor plantar response, may all be seen. If one looks carefully, however, a real profusion of signs and symptoms can often be distinguished.

These children are quite often moderately retarded in attaining physical milestones of development, particularly those requiring fine motor control. Sitting, walking, and the like, may not be much delayed, if at all; but handedness, normally clearly foreshadowed by 18–24 months, is usually delayed to the fourth or even fifth year. The child may run about freely, but riding a tricycle defies him for years, and fastening buttons may be impossible until six or seven years. Clear-cut apraxia is seldom present, but an effort to tie his shoelaces brings out a thousand frantic turnings and twistings; and hopping on one foot, a task the normal five-year-old does well, is painful to watch, so clumsily, inexpertly, and unsteadily is it done. Emotional instability is the rule. The child swings from violent aggressiveness through extreme timidity and clinging to his parents, to effusive emotionality, and back to tears—almost as he is watched. This is combined with another feature: a marked hyperactivity and distractability. These are the children who can never sit still long enough to have a story read to them; who are constantly on the go, roaming about the consulting room, peering into drawers, upsetting one's examining basket, running to the window at every sound, poking into one's pockets at one moment, and climbing onto their mothers' laps and refusing to be touched, the next.

Their physical awkwardness and unpredictable mood swing make it hard for them to find friends, and the parents almost always recount that either they have no friends at all, not infrequently because the neighbors have forbidden their own children to associate with the neighborhood outcast, or else that they can play with only a much younger child, or perhaps with a much older person.

When the parents are asked to describe what exactly the child does which is so bad, they usually are at a loss to think of anything of any moment. In the words of one fine clinician, "it is not that his behavior is so bad, it is just that there is so much of it." Questioned more closely, his mother will generally agree that when he is alone with her, he can perform quite well and is often quiet and lovable, though, even then, hyperactive and distractable to a degree. His schoolwork is poor, and he gets good marks only in those things he can, in one way or another, commit to memory. Efforts to tutor him are usually failures, especially if this involves keeping him working at one task for more than 10 or 15 minutes at a stretch.

Other difficulties may be present, the commonest ones having to do with the child's development of speech and language. These vary from slow development of infantile articulation, difficulties and substitutions in the use of connecting words and phrases, to outright aphasias. Reading difficulties are common—failure to recognize and distinguish between various words and forms, reversals, and the like; and when writing, not only these are demonstrated, but also a marked difficulty with perception of shape, form, and spatial relationships. School children of eight or nine years may have no grasp of the spatial arrangement of their script on the page, and be quite unable to copy simple geometric forms from memory, or even with the originals before them.

As noted, the physical examination of such children is unrevealing until one begins to search for evidences of early aphasia and apraxia, by the simple tests of shoelace tying, figure copying, hopping, copying of dictated material, and the like. Laboratory examinations are likewise not helpful. Dr. David Clark states: "Such children in an earlier day were regarded as possesed of original sin, or mentally retarded, or both," and explains that the tag "brain damage" is also being put on children "in whom historical evidence or physical signs to support diffuse brain injuries is lacking." "The diagnosis is an attractive one," he adds, "if for no other reason than that it removes the stigma of mental retardation from the family, and converts the child from an object of shame to one of pity and potential curability. It is at present being made far too often by educators, social workers, psychologists and the like, who have no place in the domain of organic neurological disease."

To understand the complicated process of reading and the effect brain damage may have upon it, we must look at the parts of the brain which become involved in the reading process. There are six areas of the brain which are important in the reading process.

The printed word is first seen by the eye, which serves only to form an image which is relayed to the brain for interpretation. These images are transmitted as electrical impulses from the retina of the eye to the optic nerve, and then to the occipital cortex, and finally to the area known as the area of Brodmann. Brodmann's area has three parts which are referred to as areas 17, 18, and 19. Area 17 is the first to receive the visual signal. Injury to this part of the brain may produce slow reading because of its inability to identify the written word, but not a specific reading disability. Area 18 is next to area 17 and surrounds it like a reversed letter C. This area is activated only by impulses starting in area 17 and is concerned only with visual memory patterns. It is this area which enables a child to see a chair or a cat, and to remember the visual images so that he recognizes them the next time he sees them. The upper part of area 18 functions in the recognition of animate objects, such as the cat, while the lower part acts in the recognition of inanimate objects, such as the chair. Destruction of this area results in loss of ability to recognize objects and is called visual agnosia. The ability to read, however, is not affected.

Area 19, also shaped like the letter C, surrounds area 18, and is stimulated by area 18. It is concerned with the elaboration of memory patterns necessary for the recall of animate and inanimate objects and also of language symbols. Destruction of this area results in loss of memory of things, of persons, and of language. A patient may not be able to tell how many legs a cat has, or the difference between an apple and an orange. He may also be unable to read.

The fourth area of the brain important to the reading process is called the angular gyrus. This area is connected with all of the other five, and is essential in both reading and writing.

Injury to the angular gyrus will cause a person to be unable to read. The patient sees the printed word but cannot interpret it.

Another area of importance in the reading process is the area of Wernicke, concerned with the recognition and recall of speech. Since there are nerve connections between Wernicke's area and the angular gyrus, and since this area reinforces the ability to understand written language by auditory stimulation, or by hearing the word, it comes into play in the learning process when the teacher speaks a word and asks the child to repeat what is heard.

The final area of the brain that could be of importance is the area of Broca, which is also connected with the angular gyrus and is concerned with the motor function of speech. Its function is demonstrated by those individuals whose silent reading is associated with lip movement. In these cases the visual image stimulates the muscles which have to do with speaking, demonstrating the close connection between the visual and speech areas of the brain.

Injury in either Wernicke's area or the area of Broca can complicate the learning process, especially when the educator and reading therapist use classroom techniques which involve hearing the spoken word and repeating what is heard.

If there should be a lesion in the left occipital lobe and another lesion in the splenium of the corpus collosum, no impulses from the primary visual areas can reach the left angular gyrus. The person thus affected therefore suffers from *alexia without agraphia* (agraphia meaning the inability to write). So, alexia without the inability to write occurs when there is a lesion in the angular gyrus of the left cerebral hemisphere. Alexia alone occurs when there is a lesion in the angular gyrus plus a lesion in the corpus collosum. A child who suffers from dyslexia may be able to recognize letters if he traces them with his finger or if someone holds his finger and traces letters with it. This is due to the fact that the impulses originating in the parietal cortex of the brain, which bring kinesthetic information from the tracing finger, are sent to the angular gyrus where decoding impulses of visual, auditory, and kinesthetic origin have been encoded and previously memorized. Therefore, the dyslexic child may have lost his ability to recognize words or letters, but he can still see and write spontaneously.

Masland[40] has done a thorough study of the complex brain mechanisms and neurological functions underlying the language function.

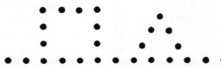

Figure. 1.   Although in reality this is only a series of dots, when viewed, it conveys the perceptual configuration of a square and a triangle.

Perception and visual interpretation is another important part of reading which should be understood. This involves the *Gestalt* phenomenon and consists of a putting together of the visual impulses. In Fig. 1 is a series of dots. The normal brain does not perceive them as a series of isolated dots, but rather as a square and a triangle sitting on a line. Thus the brain perceives these dots as organized into a configuration.

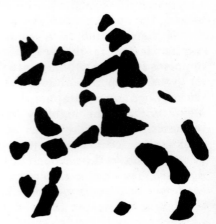

Figure. 2.   Man on Horseback.

Figure 2 shows another series of dots. This one is more complex. Here, the normal brain will perceive the grouping of shapes as a man on horseback, possibly with some action indicated. In this case, a person who has severe brain damage will see this as merely a series of dots.

In this way the brain builds up a visual pattern. This

Gestalt phenomenon is also illustrated in reading. If a child with visual-motor disability or incoordination sees the teacher flash a word on the board, he will not be able to see it as a complete word, but only as a series of letters without meaning.

For quite some time brain damage has been suspected of being a cause of learning disability, but modern concepts of minimal brain dysfunction have developed only recently. The incidence of learning disabilities is more frequent than the combined total of mental retardation, cerebral palsy, and epilepsy. In 1947, Strauss and Lehtinen[41] wrote an excellent book on the psychopathology and education of the brain-injured child, stressing the psychological drawings of children suspected of brain damage.

An interesting series of cases was reported in 1959 by Kawi and Pasamanik.[42] These men studied the records of 205 children who had reading problems. It was found that 16.6% of them had been exposed to two or more complications during birth or immediately thereafter. Records of a similar group of children without reading problems revealed that only 1.5% of this group had complications at birth.

Kawi and Pasamanik concluded that the complications encountered by these children at birth were such that they might cause some degree of lowered oxygen content to the brain (fetal anoxia). Since the blood vessels to the part of the brain which is concerned with reading ability are terminal end vessels, this area is the first to be affected by a lack of oxygen to the brain. They reported that severe cases of fetal anoxia result in miscarriage, stillbirth, spontaneous abortion, and neonatal death. Less serious forms of injury lead to cerebral palsy, and epilepsy, while very minor injury leads to behavior problems, speech disorders, and retarded reading. This report was one of the first indications in modern research that there was a neurological condition associated with dyslexia or learning disability.

Gesell, an authority in the field of education, in writing about the development of children, has also expressed the belief that unrecognized minimal birth injury may express itself in speech difficulty and may later appear in the form of reading difficulty. In studies of such children he found them to be clumsy; they could not button their shirts, had poor hand-and-eye coordination in bouncing a ball, and showed general muscular incoordination.

The statement has been made that the "continuum" of Kawi and Pasamanik is to be doubted because in premature children there is a higher incidence of brain damage, and yet there is no higher incidence of prematurity in dyslexia. This is not unusual, since in cerebral palsy there is a global damage to the brain; in dyslexia the changes are minimal and may exist with no manifest organic lesion. The changes may be genetic, resulting from altered molecular protein synthesis. So the relationship of brain damage to prematurity does exist, but the implication of prematurity to learning disabilities does not necessarily follow.

An analogy to this is the fact that the more frequently there are ocular findings in cerebral palsy, the more severe is the mental retardation.[43] Similarly, the less severe the mental retardation, the less severe the ocular defects. So, by analogy, the more extreme the prematurity, the more severe the brain damage. The less extreme the prematurity, the less severe the brain damage.

Following the study by Kawi and Pasamanik, a report was published by Walsh and Lindenberg[44] that discussed the damage to optic nerve pathways which occurred when the child suffered from hypoxia, or lack of oxygen. It was their contention, agreeing with Kawi and Pasamanik, that children could suffer from varying degrees of hypoxia and perinatal distress. It was the conclusion of both groups that if there was a considerable oxygen lack, there could be abortion or the child could be stillborn. With less severe degrees of oxygen lack, the child would perhaps suffer from epilepsy or cerebral palsy, and with minimal degrees of hypoxia or oxygen lack, a less severe neurological impairment could result in the child developing speech difficulties or learning disabilities.

Other research soon demonstrated the possibility of neurological handicaps in another way. This related to the finding that some children cannot reproduce geometric designs. They cannot copy a box or a triangle, or draw a flag. This finding accorded with the Bender-Gestalt Test, which reveals that children with brain damage show some inability to produce meaningful geometric forms. This difficulty in drawing geometric forms and the inability to perform successfully the Bender-Gestalt Test is further evidence of cerebral dysfunction and has become evidence for part of a symptom complex associated with soft neurological signs. In 1962, Richmond Payne[45] discussed the minimal chronic brain syndrome in children, while Prechtl and Stemmer[46] emphasized the prominence of choreiform movements (a wide variety of rapid, jerky, but well-coordinated and involuntary movements) as a symptom of minimal brain damage.

Among other diagnostic procedures, the psychological tests are of great value. A personalized WISC will contribute the most to our understanding of a reading disability. There is a very great variation or scatter in the WISC scores. There may be a variation by as much as 15 to 20 points. Frequently, it is the performance part of the WISC that is most significant and most affected in neurological dysfunction.

The diagnosis of possible brain damage can be assisted by taking a careful medical history of the child. The mother may have had some complications of pregnancy before or during birth, such as cyanotic spells or perhaps a convulsive seizure. Postnatal brain damage might have resulted from dehydration or head injury. Perhaps there was a high bilirubin level at birth, or there may have been a low birth weight.

Tests of perception provide our most positive evidence for making a diagnosis of minimal brain dysfunction. There are a number of tests which are helpful, including that of matching geometric designs or the figure-ground discrimination test suggested by Werner and Strauss.[47] Critchley[48] identifies astereognosis as a sign that is associated with abnormalities of the parietal lobes of the brain. This is an inability to recognize objects by their shape when feeling them with eyes closed.

In 1964, Birch and Belmont[49] devised a test which involved the matching of Morse Code signals to printed dots or dot-dash combinations. This is a test of short-term memory. Another test of immediate memory involves digit repetition, or the ability of the child to repeat sequences of numbers backward and forward. This ability is often quite poor in children who have minimal brain dysfunction but who, by contrast, may also have a good memory for facts or the ability to memorize in general. Obviously, both attention and motivation affect the results of this digit test.

Also, in the minimal-brain-dysfunction group, a test of praxis (action of command performance) frequently will reveal some impairment. This involves the drawing of a geometric design from memory or the ability to place furniture or reproduce a floor plan of a familiar room.

A frequent sign of organic dysfunction, characterized as a "soft sign," is the child's inability to button his shirt or to tie his shoes. In some cases of minimal brain dysfunction, there is an impairment of the ability to perceive figures traced on the skin with a blunt instrument (graphaesthesia).

Further evidence of neurological damage appeared around 1967. Ali Khoudadoust[50] studied 1000 children who had been born at the Baltimore City Hospital. He took pictures of the backs of their eyes (fundus photography) and found that 25% of these children had evidence of retinal hemorrhages. (See Fig. 3). A survey of existing literature revealed three other medical studies which also reported a 25% incidence of hemorrhages in the retina of the newborn. Further analysis of these figures showed that, if the mother had had no previous children (primipara), there was a 39% chance of the child having retinal hemorrhages. If, however, the mother was multiparous (having had children before), the frequency of retinal hemorrhages dropped to approximately 21%. In other words, there is ample existing evidence of retinal hemorrhages in newborn children. These findings suggest that there is a possibility that some damage may be done to the child's central nervous system at birth as he passes through the birth canal.

Other evidence of brain damage lies in electroencephalo-

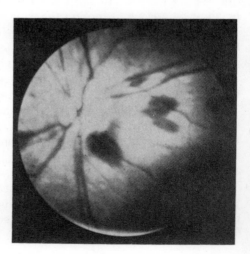

Figure 3. Retinal hemorrhages in newborn infant in the first 48 hours of life.

graphic (EEG), or brain-wave, studies done by the author on 100 children. Fifty of these children had severe degrees of reading disability but no overt signs of neurological damage. When the EEG tracings of a control group of 50 normal children were compared to the group of dyslexics, the children with severe learning disabilities registered a higher instance of EEG abnormalities. The EEGs of all 100 cases were analyzed in a double-blind study. Interpretations were done independently, by someone who had no knowledge of the clinical history and the results were determined. Using special techniques, abnormalities were detected in 40 of the 50 students who were retarded readers, and in only 7 of the 50 in the control group who were reported to be normal.[51]

Although brain-wave tracings can be reported accurately only by a highly trained neurologist, it is important to understand what the electroencephalograph is and how it works. The brain sends out waves of energy, much the same as a radio or television transmitter sends out waves, except that the brain waves are only by-products of what is going on inside. And, like smoke from a factory chimney, they give only a general indication of what is actually going on inside. For example, it is not possible to relate specific thoughts to specific EEG patterns.

Electrodes are placed on different parts of the head. These are pieces of metal acting as conductors. They pick up the waves being transmitted from the particular parts of the brain nearest to them. These waves are passed into the machine and amplified; they then are traced onto the moving graph paper as a permanent record of the wave pattern being given off. These patterns indicate whether the brain is functioning normally or whether there is damage present in any particular area. A sudden discharge, wave slowing, or lack of wave activity from any area may indicate injury or disease.

Figure 4 shows such a graph, recorded from a person with normal wave activity. The lines are fairly regular in pattern. The normal rhythm is generally 8–13 cycles per second. The top four lines record the right side of the brain, and the lower four lines the left hemisphere. (Numerous other combinations are possible, however.) There is a definite similarity between the two.

Now compare these with the recordings of a retarded reader who shows no other signs of brain damage (Figure 5).

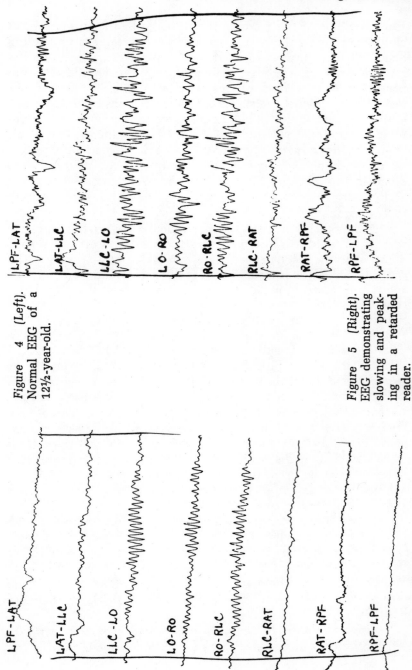

Figure 4 (Left).
Normal EEG of a
12½-year-old.

Figure 5 (Right).
EEG demonstrating
slowing and peak-
ing in a retarded
reader.

Ettlinger has reported 10 cases of adult patients with brain damage in area 19 of Brodmann. Careful examination of the visual-motor functions of these patients showed that they could copy very simple designs but were unable to represent perspective—such as a cube; and drawings from memory showed characteristic disarticulation and piecemeal procedure. Designs were poorly copied and in some cases the patient was even slow and awkward in tying knots, often being satisfied with mere twists of the string. Furthermore, examinations with the Wechsler-Bellevue test gave results indicating an average or high intelligence level. A striking note of similarity with his cases to ours is found in the EEG. In the normal individual, symmetrical parts of the brain produce waves which are alike. In Ettlinger's tracings, however, the two are not symmetrical, and indicate damage to one side of the brain.

Penfield,[52] a neurosurgeon from Montreal, operated on 17 patients who had focal epilepsy as a result of brain damage involving the parietal occipital area. He gave these patients IQ tests and visual-motor tests, and also did routine brain wave tracings, both before and after operation. The test results showed that these patients had suffered no impairment of intellectual capacity. The EEGs showed abnormalities such as we found with retarded readers, and visual-motor disturbances appeared which were the same as those found in other cases of retarded readers.

Electroencephalograms had been performed on reading-retarded children before, but never under these rigid conditions of testing. Margaret Kennard,[53] for example, performed EEGs on retarded readers from a psychiatric ward. She found abnormalities in nearly 80% of the cases, but it is well-known that the brain wave tracings may be abnormal if the patient is in a psychotic state. Another example is that of Dr. Taylor Stratten of the Montreal Children's Hospital, who studied routine brain wave tracings of 950 patients. In those which were abnormal, he found a high percentage of children with reading problems. It must be emphasized that the EEG is only one of a battery of tests which assist the physician in making a diagnosis. In itself, it is not diagnostic and must be considered as only one of many findings.

Many such cases could be cited to show the similarities between reactions of patients with known brain damage and the retarded readers. The question we must ask now is, "what causes such slight brain dysfunction?" No one has the answer to this exactly. The brain is of course extremely complicated, and there is much about its functioning we do not know.

Thus far we have mentioned the positive EEG findings, the failure to do geometric drawings, the historical studies of Kawi and Pasamanik, the studies of Walsh and Lindenberg—all of which have suggested a strong bias toward the presence of cerebral dysfunction. But there remain other investigations that are even stronger in their indication of the presence of possible brain dysfunction as a cause of learning disabilities.

The studies of Khoudadoust contained children who had no history of perinatal distress and were routine births. What happens to these children when they begin school? A small but inconclusive group of these children, re-examined at the age of seven years, were found to be normal. But is this the group that develops speech problems and learning disabilities?

Another strong bit of evidence was published by Towbin[54] in the Journal of the American Medical Association in August, 1971. He demonstrated cerebral and cortical damage in children who had varying degrees of hypoxia. He actually demonstrated histological evidence of cortical atrophy in these children who had suffered from hypoxia. These two additional studies, when combined with the previous evidence noted above, provide convincing evidence that damage to the brain, either major or minimal, and even only chemical, can produce a dysfunction that would result in a learning disability.

It has been established that experience, including the experience of learning, alters the chemistry of the brain. In fact, it is suggested that the act of learning itself sets in motion a process that alters the protein-RNA structure of the brain. Experiments with rats have shown that injections of certain drugs appear to enhance learning and long-term memory, while others seem to suppress or enhance short-term memory without affecting long-term memory. While conceding the extreme complexity of the learning process, this research suggests that mental retardation is not a single phenomenon, but perhaps due to defects in specific and discrete areas of the brain. While the implications of this research must remain extremely tentative for education and the treatment of human beings, at least one scientist[55] has suggested that an arsenal of drugs may soon be developed whereby the intellectual capacity of children, perhaps even adults, can be altered. While there is no agreement now on this possibility, the on-going studies of the learning process and of brain chemistry suggest that some learning disabilities today may be the product of minimal chemical imbalances in the brain.

Hormonal abnormalities have been identified with cerebral maldevelopment. If treatment is not begun before the age of one year, severe brain damage will result. But even with treatment or minimal treatment, unrecognized forms of the deficiency could result in learning disabilities of a specific nature.

Diagnosis of the deficiency state is the responsibility of the pediatrician, who should suspect it. Hyperthyroidism can produce a period of hyperactivity and a deterioration of school work. Children diagnosed as hyperthyroid are most often initially referred to the physician because of a change in work habits and attitudes.

Pancreatic disease can cause hyper- and hypoglycemia. Frequent attacks of hypoglycemia can lead to severe mental retardation. The deficit is due to lack of nourishment to the brain as a result of the attacks. The younger the child, the more susceptible is the brain to damage. It is possible in rare cases that other endocrine glands could cause some deviation in cerebral development, but these are isolated cases and have little significance in specific learning disabilities.

Malnutrition prior to birth can cause alterations in skeletal size and cerebral development. The malnutrition which is more often associated with learning disabilities is not the type that affects the development but the social performance of the child because of his preoccupation with his immediate needs.

With reference to the early detection of neurological abnormalities in newborn infants, the serum bilirubin levels and low birth weight are important indicators. Routinely studying the bilirubin levels of a large number of newborns, Hardy and Peeples[56] found that 84% had maximum levels below 10 milligrams percent; 5% had bilirubin levels of 15 or above, and 2% had levels of 20 or more. They also noted that babies weighing 1500 grams or less, and those born after less than 37 weeks of gestation, had significantly higher levels of serum bilirubin than the larger, more mature infants. Comparisons have been made between a control group of full-term infants, and there were significantly more deaths in the neonatal period in children with high bilirubin levels than among the control group. There was also a significant difference in the intelligence levels of the two groups.

As we have seen, the maturing brain, both before and after birth, may suffer damage that ultimately results in an impairment of neurologic function. This damage may result not only in the *reduction* of the function of the central nervous system but also in an *aberration* of function.

The cause of minimal brain dysfunction has been linked to environmental influences, heredity, nutrition, toxicity, endocrine, and other processes. Birch[57] set forth in 1964 an excellent review of the various problems related to brain damage in children. He pointed out that brain damage can vary with respect to its origin, extent, location, type of lesion, duration of damage, the rate at which the damage has been sustained, and the time of life or developmental stage at which the injury has occurred. But Birch stated that the evidence was still poor for concluding that children who exhibit the behavioral pattern do, in fact, have damage to the brain.

At that time, Birch was essentially correct regarding the available evidence. The relationship of learning disability to brain damage was a hypothesis and was received with caution by some people, with skepticism by others. This writer has always felt that there was a percentage of children who had some minimal brain damage. This view was based upon the results of studies done on perinatal histories, psychological drawings, the EEG tracings, frequent evidence of retinal hemorrhages in the newborn, and, clinically, the child with a normal or higher than average IQ, but with a specific disability with reference to his intelligence testing.

Now we have the first real proof of brain injury that is of such marginal intensity that gross neurological findings are not evident, but are sufficient to produce the so-called minimal brain dysfunction. Towbin has been able to study neuropathological material received at the Harvard University Medical School and has collected over 600 neonatal case studies. He has demonstrated that four main forms of cortical and spinal damage occur in the human fetus and the newborn. These four forms are: (1) subdural hemorrhage caused by traumatic dural venous tears, (2) spinal cord and brain stem damage because of mechanical injury at birth, (3) oxygen-lack damage to the deep cerebral structures which occur mainly in the premature child, and (4) hypoxic damage to the cerebral cortex in the mature fetus and the newborn child. The resulting injury depends upon two factors: (1) the severity of the episode of oxygen lack, and (2) the location of the lesion in the brain.

Pathologically, Towbin found two consistent factors. Some of the lesions showed persistent hemosiderin which is the consequence of a previous hemorrhage, and, secondarily, demonstrated glial scarring. Another type of lesion has been shown, described as ischemic neuronal necrosis. This is a condition where there is an ultimate decrease of neurons in the brain. This can inhibit or distort proper brain function, but the decrease of neurons is so lightly distributed that it escapes detection even when the tissue is examined microscopically. A loss of up to 30% of cells may go unrecognized even by an experienced neuropathologist. This type of loss of cellular elements of the brain, although not visible anatomically, may be associated with significant disability in a child.

The hypothesis of minimal brain damage—which had been previously suggested by psychological drawings, EEG changes, clinical findings of hyperactivity and poor attention span, the presence of hemorrhages in 25% of the newly born, and clinical birth histories of damage—has now been provided with more conclusive evidence. Towbin's work offers the first *pathological* criteria to show that *there is* a syndrome called "minimal brain dysfunction," and that there is positive histological evidence by which a child would be placed in that category.

In the period from 1960 to approximately 1965, there was a great tendency for those involved in learning to indiscriminately use the label "brain damage"; the label was an ugly one, and it created a sense of apprehension and despair in both parents and teachers, so that it was decided that the use of it had gone too far. This diagnostic term was therefore generally dropped from the educator's vocabulary. A host of other names were then applied to the problem, including minimal brain damage, minimal cerebral dysfunction, minimal chronic brain dysfunction or syndrome, or special education difficulties—all synonymous with "brain damage." "Minimal cerebral dysfunction" is perhaps the least objectionable because it lacks the objectionable words "damaged" or "injured." The latter two words imply to parents a situation of futility, and they provide teachers with a reason for failure which could result in diminished motivation of the teacher who attempts to teach the child.

It is very important to avoid thinking that all children who have symptoms that have been identified previously as being minimally brain-damaged, are actually brain-damaged. There is also a group of children known as immature or "late bloomers." These are children who exhibit some immaturity at the period between six and eight years of age. Not every child who begins school at the age of six is actually ready for the school experience. Children who are immature should not be exposed to the regular learning experience because it can be traumatic and frustrating.

The evidence for immaturity is drawn from two definite areas. On the "Draw-a-Person" test, there is an observable maturational lag in the immature child's drawings. Another significant finding lies in the fact that if x-rays are taken of the small bones of the child's feet and hands, a visible maturational lag is perceivable. In six-year-olds, there is an almost 2-year difference between boys and girls. This is because the growth centers of the small bones of the hand and feet (the metacarpals and metatarsals) tend to ossify at a much earlier age in the female than in the male. For instance, in a six-year-old girl there is a 2-year difference in the ossification of the greater multangular wrist bone when compared with that of a six-year-old boy. These maturational differences may account for the reading readiness of some and the lack of readiness of others at the same age. Hence the latter, whose rate of maturation is slower, are often called "late bloomers." To call these children "brain-damaged" would be erroneous. If they are recognized, properly protected, and properly taught, these "immature children" will succeed (and could even be superior) at a later age.

Parents constitute a part of the problem of managing children with brain dysfunction. Most of them are unable to accept the fact that their children do have some sort of deficiency. Therefore, our society is full of parents who are working overzealously in the field of learning disabilities because their children have "dyslexia." This word is easier for a parent to accept than the term "brain damage." This is a very disconcerting problem. It makes the formula for teaching children with brain dysfunction extremely difficult because some of them should have altered goals of achievement. Yet, the parents who want to accept the word "dyslexia" are not going to be very happy when it later becomes very clear that the child's failure to acquire knowledge is really due to brain damage or perhaps a low intellectual capacity.

In the last five years educators and parents properly have rebelled against the label of brain damage. Such a diagnosis implied too harsh a prognosis and one which frequently was not merited. The label brain damage often gave the educator and child a feeling of futility which frequently resulted in a failure of motivation. Appropriately, the word "dysfunction" should be used but the evidence is sufficient to imply that this dysfunction may be due to central nervous system damage of a limited type. It is very important that there be communication with parents so that they will have a better understanding of the educator's problem in dealing with the child who has a specific learning disability, especially if brain damage is a possible etiological factor.

Not only is the parent to be considered, but the teacher must be made aware of the fact that his or her responsibility is still to teach. No matter what the origin of the reading retardation might be, he or she cannot just give up on the child. The teacher should accept the greater challenge to understand the problem, and to teach around it. Often the child has attributes and capabilities equal to or far beyond his years. If they can be discovered, attention should be directed toward these areas of proficiency.

An excellent review of such special education has been done by Cruickshank[58] in the so-called Syracuse Study. This was one of the early efforts to set up and to evaluate different types of special-education programs. Obviously, these programs belong to the realm of the special educator. However, a word of admonition is certainly in order with reference to educational therapy. There are many diagnostic instruments and numerous instructional approaches which have come upon the scene as a result of the necessity for remedial teaching. A trial of any individualized or special-educational approach must always have a feedback of information concerning the response of the child to the individualized program. Unless there is controlled feedback or evaluation of a specific program, classification of the program is meaningless. The proliferation of new programs and systems is at best wasteful (and can be harmful) unless coupled with sound evaluations of their success.

From the medical point of view, the management of those children who have a specific learning disability due to brain damage is rather limited. Certainly acute intoxication, such as lead poisoning, should be eliminated. Metabolic diseases ought to be eliminated, and of these the phenylketonuria (PKU) and aminoacidurias in some atypical form must be considered. Intracranial lesions such as a subdural hematoma, or post-encephalitis, should be investigated, especially when the onset of the reading disability has been sudden.

Where none of these factors are involved, the medical aspect is limited. Aside from assisting in the drug therapy that is involved in the treatment of some of these children for their hyperactivity, the pediatrician's goal will be to communicate and counsel with others who are working with the child. He should act as a liason between the family, the educator, and the psychologist. This may be his most important function in the child who has reading difficulty when the etiology is classified as brain damage or cerebral dysfunction.

Medical science does not now have all the answers to the question of what causes congenital abnormalities in children, but there has been an increasing awareness of these disorders. To help find some of the answers, a gigantic research project has been inaugurated in the United States which is bringing 40,000 women and their babies under the watchful eyes of medical researchers over a period of at least 5 years, in 16 medical institutions throughout the country.

The study has been organized by the National Institute for Neurological Diseases and Blindness, a research arm of the U.S. Public Health Service, which will coordinate the work of these medical centers. Because a great number of factors can adversely affect a child during pregnancy, research begins during the early stages of pregnancy. Mothers are interviewed by psychologists and examined regularly by obstetricians. Exhaustive records are compiled. During the period of labor, each mother is watched carefully, and such things as pulse, blood pressure, temperature, and fetal heart rate are recorded. During the actual delivery a pediatrician records everything that happens, since some defects result from occurrences at birth. Within minutes after the birth, the pediatrician begins his examination of the baby, checking heart rate, color, respiration, and muscle response.

The next examination of the baby takes place 1 hour later, and several other thorough examinations are made during the infant's stay in the hospital nursery. Such examinations continue, and when the child is 18 months old he is given an EEG to detect any changes that can be developmental or the result of brain damage.

This research will undobutedly answer many of the questions which exist today concerning congenital abnormalities, and may lead to new hope for children. Certainly, this information will be of great value in uncovering the underlying causes of reading retardation. The evidence of brain damage in cases of retarded readers is convincing. It is important that the educator and parent be aware of this group of children so that remedial training can be instituted at an earlier age, and "reading readiness" be more firmly established before the process of teaching reading is begun.

Medical centers involved in the National Institute for Neurological Diseases & Blindness Research project: Children's Hospital, Buffalo, N.Y.; Boston Lying-In Hospital; Boston Children's Medical Center; Brown University; Yale University School of Medicine; Columbia Presbyterian Medical Center; rological Diseases and Blindness Research project: Children's Hospital, Philadelphia, Pa.; The Johns Hopkins Hospital; Medical College of Virginia Hospital, Richmond, Va.; Charity Hospital, New Orleans, La.; University of Tennessee Medical School; University of Minnesota; University of Oregon School of Medicine; and San Francisco Children's Hospital.

The Role of Vision in Learning: Peripheral and Perceptual Factors

The average person has a number of misconceptions about the eye. In reality, it is one of the most adaptable structures of our bodies. You are not likely to injure your eyes simply by reading. You may read in glare or in the dimmest light, or you may watch television in a dark room for days on end, and although it may provoke fatigue and give evidence of eye strain, it cannot possibly injure your eyesight. Let us take a brief look at the construction of the eye and the process of vision as it functions in the act of reading.

The eye consists of a transparent covering called the cornea. Inside of this is the iris, which gives an eye its color. The dark pupil in the center of the iris is a circular space, and is dark only because there is no light inside the vitreous cavity. Behind the iris is the lens which is also transparent, and shaped somewhat like a flattened sphere. It is suspended by a web of fine ligaments and is capable of changing shape in order to focus on distant or near objects.

The center of the eyeball is filled with vitreous humor, a fluid which is 99% water and makes up most of the eye's volume. This viscous jelly helps hold the eye's shape and keep the retina in place. The retina is a transparent tissue, a paper-thin, upside-down carpet covering most of the inside of the eye.

When this covering is stimulated by light, it registers a chemical change. Light rays from any point outside the eye are bent as they pass from the air through the cornea and into the liquid aqueous humor. The rays are focused on the retina by the lens and cornea. The retina is covered with some 6½ million tiny cones which are sensitive to color, and about 120 million rods which are color-blind but are more sensitive to light than the cones.

From the retina, electrochemical impulses convey the stimulus to the brain almost instantaneously. The frequency of the impulses is what tells us how bright the light is. Dim light causes less than eight impulses per second in a nerve. Very bright light may run at up to 130 impulses per second in a nerve. Although the function of the eye can be compared with a camera, the retina is not like a photographic plate in that it registers only a temporary chemical change, which disappears in about one-tenth of a second.

If everything that has been mentioned to this point were functioning properly, one still could not read unless the eyes could move constantly and quickly, every tenth of a second. This eye movement is controlled by a set of six muscles. Our eyes are constantly moving, sweeping across the object of our focus that interests us with micronystagmoid fixations. Since the image on the retina lasts for only about one-tenth of a second, we do not notice the jerkiness. The eyes move in tandem, like the front wheels of a car, and also in opposition—to see close objects. Sharp images of objects must be formed no matter what their distance. For this purpose the lens is pliable and often changes its shape. This ability is known as accommodation, and the extent to which the eye can perform this task is defined as accommodative power or amplitude.

But beyond the mechanical functioning of the eye, the process of seeing is not complete until what is seen is interpreted by the observer. This is called *perception* and is an interpretation which is based on past experience. This is entirely a function of the brain.

Far too much emphasis is generally placed on the importance of good vision as it affects children who have reading problems. The simple fact is that *there is no definite evidence of any relationship between peripheral visual ability and reading problems.* Yet nearly every classroom teacher (as well as many reading specialists) would like to think that when a child has a problem of reading, the correction of a visual defect, whether by the use of glasses or by the use of muscle exercises, will be a substantial aid to solving the reading problem. In fact, some highly respected reading specialists have been misled to the extent that they have suggested the use of eye exercises as a helpful aid in reading problems.

A visual defect does not mean that the visual inefficiency is causing the reading problem. Some students with extremely poor vision are excellent readers. There is no agreement at all among researchers as to the connection of any eye disorder with the ability to read, or even with scholastic achievement in other areas. Nevertheless, it is certainly in order that schools give visual screening tests to detect visual disorders and make the condition known to parents, since they may contribute to "slow reading" due to an inability to identify quickly the written symbol.

There are a number of screening tests used by schools for detection of peripheral visual defects. The most frequently used is the Snellen chart which measures visual acuity, or sharpness of vision. The test determines the smallest letter that can be read at a distance of 20 feet. A visual acuity of 20/20, which is considered normal, simply means that at 20 feet the observer can read a letter 8.86 millimeters square. An acuity score of 20/30 means that at 20 feet the smallest letter the observer can read is one that should have been readable normally at 30 feet.

Another test used is the Keystone Visual Survey which goes farther in testing depth perception and muscle balance. Such a test shows whether the eyes are working together. Some schools use a Binocular Reading test which reveals the extent to which each eye sees the print when both eyes are in use.

Still another test is made possible by the ophthalmograph. This device uses cameras to photograph the movements of both eyes simultaneously. A careful examination of the film may reveal certain patterns which can be interpreted as an indication of reading habits. The graph will show clearly the case of one eye which wanders from the print, or the condition where the eyes may have to make adjustments to find the beginning of a line of print. It demonstrates the number of fixations a child must make in order to read a line of printed material.

When something is wrong with a child's vision, it is important that the condition receive competent diagnosis and treatment because a child with poor sight will have difficulty identifying details of the printed page and might become a slow reader. In the case of poor visual acuity, the condition should be correctable by the use of glasses.

Refractive visual defects include far-sightedness (hyperopia) and near-sightedness (myopia). Normal eyes can see an image 20 feet or more away clearly when the ciliary muscles of the eyes used for focusing are relaxed. The far-sighted person has a near point of clear vision that is farther away than the person with normal vision. He cannot see a near object clearly without accommodating to focus on the object. The near-sighted person is one whose eyes can see clearly at only a short distance when the focusing muscles are relaxed. This distance may vary from a few feet to as short a distance as a few inches. Both conditions can usually be corrected with lenses. The defect known as astigmatism is one which causes objects to appear distorted. This can be caused by a defect in the curvature of the cornea or lens. The condition also can usually be corrected with lenses. These abnormalities are all connected with the eye's powers of refraction. It may be helpful at this point to consider the six muscles which control eye movement.

The most common of the muscle disorders of the eye is the condition known as strabismus. With this condition there may be a horizontal deviation, as when one eye is turned in or one eye is turned out, or a vertical deviation when one eye is turned up or down. The unused eye, as a result of suppression, may suffer from varying degrees of visual impairment. This may result in a condition called amblyopia ex anopsia. Glasses help in many cases—but not in others. Others of these cases can be helped with surgery, during which the deviating eye is moved to the correct position.

To illustrate how reading specialists are often mislead by misunderstandings about eye exercises, or "visual training" as it is called, the following case is summarized:

A patient was sent for a 10-week summer session to a *refractionist* (a specialist in visual training). The refractionist saw this student for visual training each morning, and then each afternoon the child went to the reading clinic. It was claimed that the child could use both eyes effectively at far distances, but he could read at near distance with only one eye. It was also directed that one eye be covered for a period of 15 minutes, then the other eye covered for the same length of time during the period when the child was visiting the reading clinic. After 4 weeks the reading tutor was informed that the child could use both eyes together at reading distance for ½ hour each day. Finally, the report concludes with the direction that after 6 weeks there should be no limitations on the child's reading except that he be permitted short periods of relief from near-point activities whenever he requested them. Then, during the last 4 weeks of this therapy, the relief periods became less frequent and were finally eliminated. The report concludes that as a result of this "visual training" program the child was able to improve his reading as much as any other child in the clinic.

This case is an example of the type of misdirection which is extremely dangerous, and against which reading specialists and parents must be on guard. The exercises described could not have been of any value to the child's reading, and any improvement that was noted could only have been the result of the other tutorial factors which were taking place in the afternoon reading sessions. In this case, the personal attention received by this child was probably enough to increase his motivation, thereby enabling him to improve at the same rate as others in the class. The theory of giving muscle exercises is that the eyes can coordinate better and the child can be taught better visual and perceptive habits, and thus be enabled to read better. The exercises start with teaching one eye to move freely, then the other eye to move freely. After this freedom of monocular vision has been established, the same process is attempted with both eyes working together. Then the attempt is made to improve the facility of accommodative change, that is, to develop the ability to focus freely from far to near and back again.

The procedure is called "accommodative rock." These exercises also attempt to establish stereopsis, or depth perception, for both far and near objects. They attempt to eliminate suppressions of either eye, to build fusion reserves, and establish hand-eye coordination. In addition to being expensive, it is my contention that these exercises are a waste of time as an aid to reading. The only real benefit a child might get from them is the increased motivation which will come from the attention and understanding he gets during the reading therapy.

Clinicians in centers attached to medical schools and universities are apprehensive about the almost mystical nature of certain treatment methods advised by some private remedial centers. Schools are often pressured by parents and influential board members to adopt one or another approach as an aid in teaching reading. Since many of the recommendations for treatment of learning disabilities include "eye exercises," it is important that professionals investigate some of the techniques which have been prescribed and are being used by some disciplines. One important area has to do with ocular motility in the dyslexic child.

About 1936 the ophthalmograph was developed to photograph ocular movements during reading. The machine was adequate in demonstrating ocular movements; the characteristics of the reading habit and the nature of binocular motor coordination during reading could be interpreted from the reading graph. The technique was good, but the analysis of the resulting graphs suffered from misinterpretation—it was claimed that the faulty eye movements represented on these graphs were the *cause* of poor reading.

Routine muscle tests were thought to be inferior to the ophthalmographic record because in the former the eye movements were not measured in the actual reading situation. It was thought that the muscle test created a special visual situation under which the eyes were then measured. The objection was that these relationships were interpreted in terms of a wider functional ability than the scope of the test would allow.

The relative importance of good ocular movement to good reading becomes apparent when one claims that the smoother and more accurate the binocular activity, the faster and more efficient is the reading. Inadequate understanding of this relationship and of the implications of the reading graph may re-

sult in educators suggesting orthoptic or muscle exercises in
an effort to train ocular movements, believing that this would
be beneficial in improving reading. A common practice is to
obtain the child's reading graph in the first grade, expose him
to the tachistoscope or perhaps some form of orthoptic exercise, and then retest his ocular movements at the end of the
academic session. It is claimed that improvement in ocular
motility is the reason for the child's improved reading ability.

A publication of the American Optical Company Bureau
of Visual Science (1950) claimed that various abnormalities
indicated on a series of graphs were the cause of certain cases
of reading failure. Lengthy fixations indicated slow reaction to
the printed material. It was claimed that exercise with the
tachistoscope resulted in better control of eye movements and
improved reading ability. Abnormalities of excessive convergence, it was said, resulted in a lack of rhythm in the reading
pattern and a consequently poor reading ability.

To investigate this subject, the present authors examined
the eye movements of 50 dyslexic children and an adequate
number of normal children to serve as normal controls. The apparatus used in our experiment was the electronystagmograph,
a machine which measures the difference in the electrical potential between the retina and cornea synchronous with ocular
movements. Each child was asked to read material below his
frustration level, and a graph was obtained. Then he was asked
to read material above his frustration reading level. (See Fig. 6.)
The obtained graph demonstrated abnormalities which varied
with the difficulty of the word or sentence and resulted in
changes on the graph which were synchronous with difficulties
in the reading material. (See Fig. 7.) Two additional parts of the
experiment were designed. Shadow reading—reading with the
child—was done and graphs obtained as the child read both

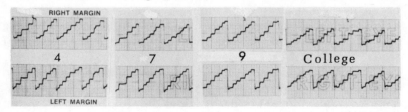

Figure 6. Normal Reader. Demonstration of normal myograph at
fourth, seventh, ninth, and twelfth year reading levels.

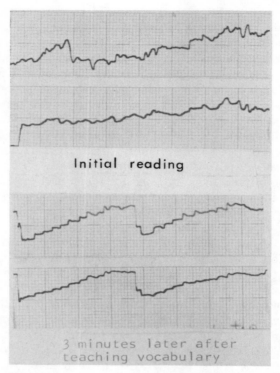

Initial reading

3 minutes later after
teaching vocabulary

Figure 7. Retarded Reader. Myograph tracings demonstrating poor reading ability (two upper tracings) and subsequent improvement in ability three minutes after vocabulary was taught.

below-frustration and above-frustration material. In all cases, the ocular movements became symmetrical and improved toward the normal pattern.

In the next experiment, the frustration words were taught in advance of reading the material. Within minutes after this previously frustrating material was read, the graph showed definite improvement over previous untutored graph recordings. In actuality, it is not the eyes that read, but it is the brain that reads. (See Figs. 8 and 9.)

In summary, the electronystagmograph and the ophthalmograph provide convenient methods for analyzing ocular movements. Findings indicate that it is the *degree of comprehension that produces the type of ocular movement*—and not ocular motility that determines the degree of comprehension. When

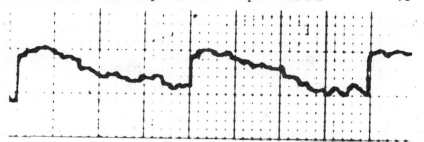

Figure 8. Japanese physician reading Japanese language material. Note normal myograph pattern.

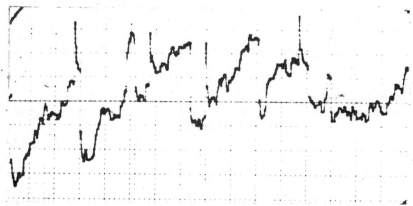

Figure 9. Japanese physician reading third grade level English. Note the irregularities in the waveform.

the child had difficulty in understanding the word or the syllable, he would exhibit regression of eye movement or often a prolonged fixation as he attempted to reconstruct the word. As soon as the child was able to understand the words, reading resumed in normal fashion. This evidence suggests that it is the ability to understand which determines the fluidity of the reading and that ocular motility simply denotes the degree of fluidity. The electronystagmograph provides a sophisticated method of studying these ocular movements. This research was done under uniocular and binocular conditions, using both the electronystagmograph and the Biometrics Eye-Trac apparatus. Improving ocular motility has become a widely discussed technique of assisting children who have learning disabilities. It has been assumed that learning difficulties in some cases were due to lack of binocular coordination. This experiment demonstrates that learning is done in the brain and not in the eyes. While the electronystagmograph and ophthalmograph do demonstrate incoordinate eye movements in children who have difficulty in reading, the experiments performed demonstrate that improper eye movements seem to be the result rather than the cause of poor comprehension.

Ocular patching, or filtration, has become a very much discussed method of stimulating learning in those children who might have crossed dominance. The following discussion will attempt to demonstrate the fallacy of such methods.

Inhibition plays a necessary and vital part in integrating a final perceptual pattern. If two similar images are presented to corresponding retinal points in each eye, the images are fused, and the final perceptual pattern is a fused single image. If the images are grossly dissimilar and are presented to corresponding points on the retina so that they cannot be fused into one perceptual pattern, one of the images is suppressed and is eliminated from consciousness. When the images are of equal stimulus, a condition of retinal rivalry exists.

If the two eyes are equal, inhibition of one macula occurs when the other occupies the focus of interest. A state of rivalry results, and the inhibition is temporary and conditioned only by use of the other eye. This occurs only during binocular activity. Either eye may function, alternately retaining good vision when in use, and reverting to perceptual blindness when the other eye does the seeing. The site of the suppression seems to be the result of a cortical inhibition.

Binocular fixation of two retinal images is the act of maintaining these images on corresponding retinal points by means of motor responses to these images (fusion movements). The most elementary type of binocularity (simultaneous perception) occurs when the two images, as seen by the two eyes, are superimposed to form one. In the second grade of binocularity there is true fusion with some amplitude, and here not only are the two images fused, but some effort is made to maintain this fusion in spite of difficulties. In the third grade (or highest type) of binocularity, the images of the two eyes are fused and are blended to produce a stereoscopic effect. This is on the perceptual level.

Patching, or filtration, is a technique in which red and green filters are used in conjunction with red and green printed material. If the green glass is over the right eye and the red glass over the left eye, the red and green material which is on the page will be alternatively neutralized and, therefore, will not be seen. Thus, we can stimulate either one eye or the other. The theory is that if the child is right-handed, right-footed, and left-eyed, an attempt is made to convert the controlling or dominant left eye to the right side, to correspond with the right-handedness and right-footedness.

There is no evidence that crossed dominance impedes learning. Both hemispheres receive visual stimuli from both eyes, and ocular dominance does not indicate that only one hemisphere is functioning. All impulses which come in by way of the right eye are actually perceived with both sides of the brain. Similarly, all impulses which come in by way of the left eye are also seen by both sides of the brain. This occurs because there is a decussation or crossing of the optic nerve fibers in the optic chiasm. Therefore, when we see with either the right or left eye, both sides of the brain are receiving sensations. If there is damage to one hemisphere, the patient will develop a hemianopsia or half visual field. This is not true in dyslexia or with any children who have reading problems.

The question should be asked, what happens to the impulse after it arrives at the occipital cortex? To demonstrate this, a simple experiment in retinal rivalry was performed. A red glass was placed over the right eye and a green glass over the left one. When a target is fixated, there is a rapid red and green alteration of stimulus as the impulse is received, first by the right eye and then by the left eye. This same phenomenon can be represented by means of a machine called the amblyoscope. If a stimulus is first presented to one eye, such as a lollipop, and another image to the opposite eye, such as the mouth of the child, the first binocularly fused image would present itself as being the lollipop in the mouth of the child. The frequency with which either stimulus is seen has nothing to do with dominance or the rate of learning.

In conclusion, parents and teachers are urged to remember how tough and adaptable the human eye is. It is impossible to injure the eye by reading or looking in any way. On the other hand, if there is an ocular defect, it should be corrected, but eye exercise will not improve one's ability to read. Eyes provide a peripheral sensory stimulus, and any normal pair of eyes does that job easily, continuously, and without conscious upkeep or care. We can assume that lack of normal vision (within limits, of course—no one can read what he can't see) is not a cause of reading problems. Poor vision may make a child a slow reader because he has difficulty identifying details, but it will not produce reversals or make him a retarded reader. Correction of the visual problem may increase speed of reading, but *it will not increase perceptive abilities.*

Optometric thought on this subject seems to be divided into two groups. Most optometrists confine their role in educational achievement to visual enhancement for the sake of clear, comfortable, and efficient visual performance. A small group follows the "developmental vision" point of view, feeling that learning in general and reading in particular are primarily visual-perceptual tasks. This group advocates "visual training" in cases of reading disability.

"Visual training" is defined by them in terms of perceptual training, but some of their therapy is directed toward peripheral training. Some of the peripheral visual abilities which are claimed to be trainable are: (1) the ability to follow smoothly and accurately with both eyes, (2) the ability to fixate quickly and accurately with both eyes on a series of fixed objects, (3) the ability to change focus quickly and without blur from far to near and from near to far, and (4) the ability to maintain attention for extended periods of time at near-point activity. In the more technical language of ocular dynamics, these abilities are classified as fixation ability, fusion, stereopsis, binocularity, and motility patterns.

Carlson and Greenspoon[59] of the Los Angeles Child Development Center have said, "we have studied much of the material provided by the optometric developmental training approach and find most of it out-dated, unsubstantiated, esoteric, and pseudo-scientific. . . . Many of the basic 'facts' it appears to accept have not stood up under close study." The reader who desires documentation for this analysis of developmental optometry should refer to the position statement at the conclusion of this chapter.

Developmental optometry, or that portion of optometrists

who advocate visual training for the treatment of learning disabilities, has performed a questionable service to child, educator, and parent. The financial sacrifice has been considerable and the value of visual training is questionable. There is no doubt that some children do improve in reading ability when visual training and tutoring are combined. But there are no adequately controlled studies that would indicate that visual training alone is correlated with an increase of reading ability. Since optometrists recognize this, it is hoped that they will come to grips with this departure from scientific procedure, and that proper, controlled research will be done before further exposing children to muscle exercises and accommodative rock.

Because it is generally agreed that peripheral factors are not causative factors in a reading disability, the developmentalists have agreed that it is not the Snellen evaluation of vision or the peripheral factors, but that it is the perceptual factors that are important. Because of its importance and uncertainty, visual perception will be discussed here in some detail. The question as to whether the teacher, psychologist, opthalmologist, pediatrician, or optometrist should have the responsibility for doing psychological tests, remains an ethical and philosophical question for each individual to decide for himself. The question as to whether perceptual training is of value remains an open question which future research will determine.[60]

The Perceptual Aspects of Vision

When a child has a reading disability, it has become common to think immediately of his eyes as a possible cause of his difficulty. Since a visual defect might contribute to slower learning, it should be corrected because reading is thus made more comfortable for the child. However, there is now general agreement that factors of visual acuity, refractive error, eye muscle imbalance, binocularity, or fusion are only peripheral and *are not causative* factors in reading disability. Many researchers have made frequent comparisons between groups of normal readers and retarded readers. None of these peripheral visual factors has been found to have a higher incidence in one group than in the other.[61-63] In fact, these investigations have proven that periphereal visual factors are irrelevant to the basic problem of reading disability and should not be considered as causes of a child's learning difficulty. Consequently, in the past few years, many educators and others interested in the field of learning have turned their attention from the eye and peripheral ocular functions as a cause of failures into the broader area of visual perception.

Anatomically, perception is the sum of what takes place from the time a visual impression is received peripherally by the eye until it is transmitted to, recorded by, and understood in the brain. This same type of stimulation is also transmitted into the brain from the areas of hearing, touch, smell, and joint positional sense. It is in the brain that all of these impulses are received, decoded, and organized so that perception and understanding take place. Because visual perception is so important in the learning and reading processes, visual perception deserves further attention.

Expressed one way, visual perception is the ability to recognize and discriminate visual stimuli and to interpret them correctly in the light of previous experiences. In another sense, visual perception is a process whereby peripheral sensory stimuli are organized in the brain. Therefore, visual perception is not an ability to see accurately but is the interpretation of what is "seen" by the brain. For example, if one looks at the four lines that form a square, a sensory impression is received on the retina of each eye. The impulses are transmitted from the retinae and are recorded in the occipital lobe of the brain. These are the peripheral visual factors which are sensory to the brain, but it is the function of the brain to recognize and understand these lines as a "square," a significant geometric form.

To use a different illustration, visual perception is a process that begins when the peripheral factors have been recorded in the occipital lobe and then transmitted to the angular gyrus of the parietal lobe. Here, an animal is perceived as a four-legged beast, and, once this has happened, it is possible to differentiate between four-legged beasts. However, it is not until the information goes through the parietal lobe to the frontal lobe of the brain that a cow or a horse can be differentiated through an understanding of their functions. This is conception or understanding. Thus, it is the brain that must provide a child with an accurate conception and understanding of what he sees.

A child may see the words **horse** and **house** on the printed page, but it is through a very complex process that the visual impression is translated and organized in the brain. Perception becomes meaningful when the child recognizes the difference in these words. Reading with understanding can take place when the child has the ability to recognize differences in words and can comprehend and understand their different meanings.

There are certain abilities which a child develops in a definite sequence, normally at certain age levels. First, there is the sensory-motor phase. This comprises the initial 18 months and constitutes that period of life when a child first becomes aware of the world around him, through movement combined with the use of all of his senses.[64] The second phase is the language phase, which begins in the second year of life. It is characterized by a rapid development of speech. Here the child learns to develop and to express ideas through speech. This is the point of the child's development where there is most apt to occur some deficit in the visual and auditory sequencing.

Following this phase of maximum language development, the maximum development of perceptual ability occurs. The perceptual phase spans the period from three-and-one-half or four years to about six years of age. Piaget refers to perception as the intuitive aspects of intelligence. Perception enables a child to recognize objects around him, directly and intuitively, without deliberation and without simultaneous use of movement. Among the abilities developing during this period are those perceptual skills necessary for discriminating two-dimensional figures. The fourth phase in the child's development, the phase of concrete operation, begins when he is about six and one-half years of age. At this point, he begins to associate his present experiences with his previous knowledge.

Visual-perceptual skills usually develop from birth to the age of six in a sequential pattern. If a child does not develop the perceptual skills before the age of six, he could have learning difficulties. It is important to know this and to be able to test children during this developmental period. For example, if

a child sees a b as a d or 24 as 42, or if, from an auditory point
of view, a child hears the correct sound but if in transferring
this sensory impression the brain receives a faulty impression,
then the child is in difficulty. His interpretation of letters and
symbols is distorted, and therefore his ability to read and correctly interpret what he reads is impaired. It is possible that
this child has a lag in the development of his perceptual skills.

There are many methods of examining a child's visual-
perception ability. The test originated by Lauretta Bender,
known as the Bender-Gestalt Test and its adaptation for use
with children, described in a book edited by Koppitz,[65] has been
one of the primary methods of investigation in the visual-
perceptual area. In the language development phase, there is
the Illinois Test of Psycholinguistic Abilities (ITPA). A principal
test for evaluation of a child's higher cognitive functions is
usually the Wechsler Intelligence Scale for Children (WISC).

Another frequently used method for examining visual perception in children is that originated by Marianne Frostig,
known as the Frostig Perceptual Tests.[66] These tests involve an
evaluation in the following areas: eye-motor coordination,
figure-ground perception, constancy of visual perception, perception of position in space, and perception of space relationships. Although the Frostig Tests for determining the
"perceptual quotient," or PQ, have been accepted enthusi-
asticly by many educators, nevertheless there has been extensive
doubt and criticism of the validity of these tests as they might
relate to reading achievement.

The study which follows was undertaken to try to evaluate
some of the theories about perception and the process of
reading.

Evaluating Perceptual Factors in Reading Disability*

"Because of these objections, and because the role of visual
perception is now so widely emphasized, reevaluation of those
areas of central cerebral organizations concerned with reading
was indicated.

"Since the act of reading involves visual memory (the ability
to recall words and meanings), visual sequencing (the seeing of

letters and syllables in proper sequence), and visual perception (the ability to detect clues for seeing the whole word or groups of words), tests that examine for these functions were used. The following tests were chosen because (1) they have been standardized, and the standardization involved all socioeconomic classes of children; (2) the tests start at a sufficiently low range of accomplishment so that all children can be included in an evaluation; and (3) the examiners had greater familiarity with the tests chosen. These examinations included:

I. Visual Sequencing
   a. Knox cubes
   b. ITPA sequencing
II. Visual Perception
   ITPA figure identification
III. Visual Memory
   Benton Visual Memory Test
IV. Reading Tests
   a. Gray Oral Test
   b. Metropolitan Reading Achievement Test
   c. Wide Range Achievement Test (WRAT)
V. Visual-Motor Tests
   Bender-Gestalt Test

"Visual sequencing was investigated by two tests. They were: (1) the Knox cubes, a test in which cubes are tapped in a definite sequence; and (2) the Illinois Test of Psycholinguistic Abilities (ITPA) tests for visual sequencing, in which tiles with designs are to be reproduced in a definite order or sequence. Visual memory was examined by means of the Benton Visual Memory Cards. In this examination a design is exposed for 10 seconds and subsequently four designs, including the one that has been exposed, are shown. The subject is expected to indicate the original design from the group. The ITPA closure or figure recognition test is a test for visual perception. The child is asked to identify as many parts of the stimulus as he can in a series of four sheets. In order to evaluate reading achieve-

*This material appeared as part of an article, "Evaluation of Visual Perceptual Factors in Reading Disability," by H. K. Goldberg and J. T. Guthrie in *Journal of Pediatric Ophthalmology*, 9:1, 18-25, 1972.[67] Reprinted by permission. (See page opposite).

ment, three reading tests were used: the Gray Oral Test, the Metropolitan Reading Achievement Test, and the Wide Range Achievement Test. Also included was the Bender-Gestalt Test for visual-motor ability.

"A score was derived from each test and the results were key-punched on computer cards. Each of the tests became a variable that was individually evaluated with respect to reading achievement.

"The purpose of the present investigation was to relate visual sequential memory and visual memory to reading in normal and disabled readers. Previous research on visual sequential memory has been either irrelevant to reading, or has been methodologically unsound as a basis for conclusions regarding reading. Silverstein, in 1962, found the Benton Test to possess fair reliability, ranging from 0.62 to 0.81, depending on the response mode. However, no correlations with reading were provided. Two studies (one by Lyle and Goyen in 1962 and one by Rizzo in 1939) have reported disabled readers to be inferior to normal readers in visual sequential memory tasks. However, both studies included tachistoscopic presentation of stimuli with exposure times of 0.1 second. Since the perceptual speed of disabled readers is known to be slower than that of normal readers, it is likely that the stimuli could not be accurately perceived by disabled readers in the short time periods used in these studies. Consequently, the alleged inferiority of disabled readers in visual memory could be attributable to a deficiency of perception. Thus, the relationship between visual sequential memory and reading has not been rigorously examined in previous investigations. In order to examine and investigate this hypothesis as to whether there is a positive correlation between visual sequential memory and reading, the present study was undertaken.

"The subjects in this study were drawn from the Baltimore City Public Schools, the Laboratory School of Towson State College, and a summer remedial program conducted at the Kennedy Institute of Baltimore, Maryland. Two groups were formed: normal readers and disabled readers. There were 81 normal readers, who had an average age of 8.55 years. The IQ of the normal group, as measured by the Weschler Intelligence Scale for Children (WISC), had a mean of 98.27, with a standard deviation of 16.07. The reading ability of this group, as assessed by the Gray Oral Test, was a grade level of 2.55, with a standard deviation of 1.93.

"The 43 disabled readers were defined as children who had an IQ score higher than 80 and reading levels two or more years behind chronological age.

"The tests of visual memory administered to all of the subjects included the Benton Visual Retention Test and the Visual Sequential Memory Test of the Illinois Test of Psycholinguistic Abilities. Both included the presentation of a series of geometric forms to the subject, the removal of the forms, and the requirement that the subject remember the forms. The response mode of the two tests is different. In the Benton, the subject is required to recognize the correct series of forms when they are presented with several incorrect alternatives. However, in the ITPA Subtest of Visual Sequential Memory, the subject is required to construct the sequence from individual forms which are available to him in the form of tiles. Other tests which were administered to the normal group were the Knox Cube Test and the ITPA Visual Closure Subtest. These tests were administered to all of the subjects individually, and the examiners did not know whether the readers were normal or disabled readers prior to the administration of the tests.

"The reading tests administered to the subjects included the Gray Oral Test, which was given to all children; the Metropolitan Reading Achievement Test, which was administered to the disabled readers; and the Wide Range Achievement Test (WRAT), which was administered to 48 of the children in the

Table II
Correlation of Visual Memory and Reading for Normal Readers

	CA	ITPAM	BVR	KCT	GO
Chronological age (CA)		0.33*	0.48*	0.39*	0.70*
ITPA Visual Sequential Memory (ITPAM)			0.38*	0.38*	0.47*
Benton Visual Retention Test (BVR)				0.34*	0.51*
Knox Cube Test (KCT)					0.34*
Gray Oral (GO)					

*p <0.01; N $= 81$.

normal group. The mean chronological age of the children who received the WRAT was 8.0 years; the mean WISC IQ was 91.42; and the mean WRAT equivalent was 2.17.

"The data were analyzed by correlating the reading test scores with the visual test scores separately for the normal and disabled readers. The results for the normal readers are summarized in Table II. The figures in the Table indicate that the performance in the Gray Oral Test correlated 0.47 with the ITPA Subtest of Visual Sequential Memory, 0.51 with the Benton Visual Retention Test, and 0.34 with the Knox Cube Test. All of these correlations were significantly greater than zero at the 0.01 level. These correlations reflect the fact that students who perform well on the Gray Oral also perform well on the three measures of visual memory, and students who perform poorly on reading also perform poorly on visual memory.

Table III
Correlation of Visual Memory and Reading for Disabled Readers

	CA	ITPAM	BVR	GO	MRC
Chronological age (CA)		0.26*	0.43*	0.59**	0.14
ITPA Visual Sequential Memory (ITPAM)			0.38*	0.15	0.12
Benton Visual Retention Test (BVR)				0.32*	0.36*
Gray Oral (GO)					0.54*
Metropolitan Reading Comprehension (MRC)					

*p <0.05; N =43.
**p <0.01.

"The relationship between visual memory and visual sequencing and reading for disabled readers is displayed in Table III. In Table IV the partial correlation coefficients as computed for all the measures of reading and visual memory are shown. The measures of visual memory and sequencing were positively correlated with the chronological ages of the subjects.

"The purpose of computing the partial correlation coefficients was to determine whether the visual tests and reading were functionally related, apart from their joint correlation with chronological age. In each case, the variable of chrono-

Table IV
Partial Correlations of Visual Memory and Reading

Tests	Normal Readers	N	Disabled Readers	N
Benton-Gray Oral	0.28**	81	0.09	43
ITPAM — Gray Oral	0.35**	81	0.17	43
Knox — Gray Oral	0.11	81	N.A.	
Benton — Metropolitan Reading Comprehension	N.A.		0.47**	43
ITPAM — Metropolitan Reading Comprehension	N.A.		0.13	43
Benton — Wide Range Achievement Test	0.47**	48	N.A.	
ITPAM — Wide Range Achievement Test	0.18	48	N.A.	
Knox Cube — Wide Range Achievement Test	0.23*	48	N.A.	

*p <0.05.
**p <0.01.
N.A. = not available

logical age was removed from the zero-order correlation co-efficients between visual memory and reading. The partial correlation is thus a pure measure of the association between reading and visual memory, statistically uncontaminated by chronological age.

"The primary outcome of the study was that the tests of visual sequential ability and visual memory were significantly correlated with several measures of reading. Some of these correlations were found to be positive and significant even after the effects of chronological age were removed from the correlations. Although a few of the significant zero-order correlations between visual memory and reading were reduced to insignificance when the effects of age were removed, the use of partial correlations rather than traditional zero-order correlations would appear to be warranted in studies of this type.

"It is particularly noteworthy that the Benton Visual Retention Test showed more of the partial correlations with reading than did all of the other tests combined. The Benton test appears to be more central to tests of reading than the ITPA Subtest of Visual Sequential Memory, and differs from the other tests in several important respects. Although all the tests re-require visual memory—that is, the tests require the examinees to remember the order of a series of stimuli presented to them—the Benton Test also requires the subject to remember both the form and the spatial attitude (rotation) as well as the sequence of the stimuli.

"The high partial correlation of the Benton Test with reading, and the moderate partial correlation of the ITPA Subtest of Visual Sequential Memory, indicate that the simultaneous operation of several memory functions is central to reading. If the coordination among these functions is disrupted, or if the functions fail to act in concert, reading is likely to be impaired. It appears that in some cases memory for form, position, or sequence may be intact when they are tested separately, but when they are tested simultanously one or more of the abilities may be inoperative. Thus, reading disability may result from the lack of coordination, interaction, and simultaneity of the several visual memory abilities required for reading. Further research into this source of reading disability appears to be promising.

"Relationships between visual sequential memory and visual memory and reading in 81 normal and 43 disabled readers were investigated. Significant, positive associations were identified between visual sequential memory and paragraph comprehension, oral reading, and word recognition. The intercorrelations of the visual memory tests were moderate, indicating that these tests do not measure identical abilities. Visual sequential memory is one of the many visual functions required for reading. Other necessary capabilities include visual perception, visual discrimination, and visual synthesis. It stands to reason that visual sequential memory depends on these three abilities. If an individual is unable to perceive a given visual stimulus—that is, if he is unable to determine whether the stimulus is present or absent—he will not be able to remember the stimulus. Similarly, if a person cannot distinguish whether two different stimuli are actually the same or different, he will not be able to retain in memory either one of the two stimuli.

"The primary outcome of the study was that visual sequential memory was significantly correlated with several measures of reading. Some of these correlations were found to be positive and significant, even after the effects of chronological age were removed from the correlations. The intercorrelations suggest that a reading disability may result from a lack of coordination among the three different visual functions required for reading: namely, visual memory, visual sequencing, and visual perception.

"The child of six and older whose perceptual-motor, visual-motor, and conceptual performance is relatively primitive is the one who is likely to run into difficulty when he is exposed to reading; based on this line of reasoning, copying tests have been done that show the effectiveness of these copying tests in screening for reading readiness, predicting school achievement, and diagnosing reading and learning problems.

"The ophthalmologist or pediatrician engaged in routine practice is not able to do highly specialized testing in the manner which is necessary in the foregoing tests. Tests such as the Bender-Gestalt and the Frostig Test should be administered by specialists trained in that field. Nevertheless, it has become important for the ophthalmologist and pediatrician to investigate central visual factors as well as peripheral factors in routine practice. In view of the objections to the Bender-Gestalt and Frostig Tests, and because of the complexity of the ITPA visual sequencing and the Benton Visual Memory Tests, investigators considered it necessary to find an easy and rapid method of studying visual perception. Their attention was directed to a copy test consisting of the nine Gesell forms. Lowder,[68] in 1956, attempted to develop an objective scoring system for these figures, similar to that developed by the authors in the present study. He then correlated the scores with "teachers' ratings" of each child's abilities. He did not control for intelligence.

"So that we could investigate further the possibilities of relating these drawing forms to reading ability, and being aware of problems of analysis in the past studies, the present study was carried out.

"The visual-motor test was a copying test composed of nine geometrical figures: circle, cross, square, triangle, divided rectangle, diamond, Greek cross, cylinder, and face-on cube. All of the figures except the Greek cross were identical to the copy forms of the Gesell Developmental Kit. Our interest was in the final drawings of the child, not in how he drew the figures, the size of the forms, or their placement on the page, all of which Dr. Gesell investigated. Thus, the stimulus figures were not printed on individual cards as in the Gesell Test, but on two 8½ x 11" pages, leaving space under each figure for the child to make his drawings.

"A group of 157 children, ages 6 years, 10 months, to 7 years, 11 months, with a mean age of 7 years, 2 months, were the participants. They were part of the Johns Hopkins Child Growth and Development Department population, participating in the Collaborative Research Project of the NINDS of the Nation Institute of Health. As a part of the Collaborative Research Project, a test battery is given to each participant when he reaches his seventh birthday. This battery includes the Weschler Intelligence Scale for Children (WISC), the Wide Range Achievement Test in Reading (WRAT), and a test of visual acuity. For a 4-month period in the summer of 1970, all participants who were given the age-seven battery were also given the visual-motor test described in this report. The mean IQ of these 157 children was 91.8 with a standard deviation of 11.9. The mean seven-year WRAT reading score was 1.64 (grade level). Participants with visual acuity of 20/70 or worse were dropped from the sample. When a participant reaches his eighth birthday, another test battery is administered. Of the 157 children, 54 had been given the eight-year battery at the time of this analysis. Included in the eight-year battery was the WRAT Reading Subtest (the same as given in the seven-year battery) and the Gray Oral Reading Test. The mean WRAT reading score was 2.44 grade level, and the mean Gray Oral score was 1.82 grade level.

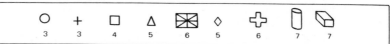

Figure 10. Gesell Figures used to correlate with reading ability at the seven-year level.

"Four criteria were identified for each figure (Fig. 10). Examples of three levels of each criterion were then found among the drawings of the participants. These became the protocols with which other drawings were compared. A well-executed criterion was given a score of 1. Thus, the score on each figure could range from 4 (a score of 1 given for each of the four criteria) to 12 (a score of 3 for each of the criteria).

Table V
Intercorrelations of Drawing, Reading, and Intelligence

	O	+	□	Δ	⊠	◇	✚	▯	⬭	Total Drawing	WRAT 7-yr.	WRAT 8 yr.	Gray 8-yr.	IQ
O		.21†	.28*	.30*	.33*	.09	.11	.22†	.17	.46*	.18	.21	.13	.07
+			.39*	.32*	.14	.13	.11	.17	.12	.45*	-.03	.10	.06	.03
□				.26*	.26*	.19	.19	.25†	.13	.51*	.06	.20	.10	.11
Δ					.36*	.24†	.38*	.28*	.29*	.63*	.26*	.39*	.28†	.26†
⊠						.36*	.44*	.29*	.39*	.70*	.28*	.21	.07	.42*
◇							.32†	.14	.27*	.56*	.33*	.36†	.21	.44*
✚								.49*	.40*	.70*	.24†	.38†	.24	.27*
▯									.30*	.58*	.20†	.40†	.26	.20†
⬭										.62*	.20†	-.06	-.11	.19
Total Drawing											.33*	.39*	.22	.41*
WRAT 7 yr.												.93*	.78*	.55*
WRAT 8 yr.													.92*	.65*
Gray 8 yr.														.49*
IQ														

*p <0.01.
†p <0.05.

Figures which were not drawn were given a score of zero.

"To check the reliability of the criteria, two scorers independently rated one figure drawn by 20 participants. Agreement of 75% was reached; that is, on 15 of the 20 figures the scorers arrived at the same total score. This was considered sufficiently high to continue the scoring procedure.

"Scores for every criterion of each figure and intelligence and reading data for each child were put on IBM computer cards. A 14 x 14 correlation matrix showed a variety of statistically significant relationships (Table V).

"All of the copying figures correlated significantly with the total drawing score, indicating that each figure contributed in some positive degree to the overall copying performance.

"The circle, cross, and square, considered to be the easiest of the forms, did not correlate with any of the three reading tests or with intelligence. This is probably because they were too easy to be able to distinguish differences in performance.

Table VI
Means and Standard Deviations of Drawing,
Reading, and Intelligence

	Mean	Standard Deviation	N
Circle	9.78	1.12	156
Cross	9.50	1.14	156
Square	8.77	1.31	156
Triangle	9.16	1.47	155
Dividend Rectangle	8.07	1.96	156
Diamond	9.04	1.79	154
Greek Cross	8.28	1.92	136
Cylinder	8.94	1.56	134
Face-on Cube	6.45	1.82	130
Drawing Total (proportion)	0.73	0.08	157
WRAT (7-year)	1.64	0.77	157
WRAT (8-year)	2.44	1.42	46
Gray Oral (8-year)	1.82	0.81	54
IQ	91.8	11.9	156

The remaining six figures were all significantly correlated with the seven-year WRAT Reading Subtest. The triangle, divided rectangle, and diamond were significant at $p < 0.01$; and the Greek cross, cylinder, and face-on cube were significant at $p < 0.05$.

"One hundred fifty seven children, ages 6 years, 10 months, to 7 years, 11 months, were given a visual-motor (copying) test composoed of nine geometrical figures. Reading tests were administered at seven years (WRAT) and eight years (WRAT and Gray Oral), and IQs were measured by the WISC at seven years. The mean IQ of the 157 children was 91.8. The mean seven-year WRAT score was 1.64 (grade level); the mean eight-year WRAT was 2.44; and the mean Gray Oral was 1.82 (Table VI). Copy tests were scored on the basis of four criteria for each of the figures, with a score of 3 indicating that the criterion was well-executed; 2, meaning fairly well-executed; and 1 meaning poorly executed. A score on each figure ranged from 4 to 12. A score of zero was given for figures not attempted. The correlation of overall drawing scores with a seven-year WRAT was 0.33, and with the eight-year WRAT, 0.39, both a $p < 0.01$. The figures which showed significant correla-

Table VII
Perceptual Ability and Reading Achievement

	IQ	WRAT (7 yr)	WRAT (8 yr)	Gray Oral
Circle	0.0675	0.1910	0.2588	0.1688
Plus	0.0324	−0.0455	0.0420	0.0167
Block	0.1138	0.0750	0.2451	0.0907
Triangle	0.2626	0.3018	0.4188	0.1236
Flag	0.4214	0.3170	0.2856	0.0184
Diamond	0.4368	0.3795	0.4784	0.0886
Cross	0.2693	0.2623	0.4488	0.2509
Cylinder	0.2016	0.2107	0.4598	0.2815
Cube	0.1869	0.2402	0.0000	0.1211

$R > 0.254$, $P < 0.01$; $R > 0.321$, $P < 0.001$; where $N > 100$.

tiions with reading at seven years were the triangle, divided rectangle, and diamond ($p<0.01$), and the Greek cross, cylinder, and face-on cube ($p<0.05$). IQ was also significantly correlated with drawing scores at 0.41, $p<0.01$ (Table VII).

"A significant correlation has been established between visual perception, visual memory, and visual sequencing, on the one hand, and reading achievement. The intercorrelations are moderate, suggesting that a reading disability may result from a lack of coordination among these three visual functions.

"The second part of this presentation provides a rapid and simple visual perceptual task, for office use, that is correlated with reading efficiency. It is emphasized that these findings do not support the indiscriminate use of perceptual training in the treatment of learning disorders. It has been well-documented that perceptual training after the age of six years is of questionable value in the treatment of learning disorder. Time spent in the teaching of reading might accomplish greater benefits than that time spent in perceptual training. Such training could be of benefit at the ages of one to six years in the reading-readiness stage, but after this period the child makes his own compensations to residual deficits."

Insofar as the educator is concerned, this conclusion is of vital importance. Ordinarily, when a teacher finds a child with a visual-perceptual deficit, the teacher will begin to work on that area of perception by various techniques. One of the commonest forms of treatment is that called the Fernald Technique or, as it is usually shortened, VAKT. This stands for Vision, Auditory, Kinesthetic, and Tactile training. What Grace Fernald[69] advocates is that, if a child is deficient in vision, then train him by the auditory, kinesthetic, and tactile methods. Or, if he is deficient in auditory perception, then train the child with emphasis upon the visual, tactile, and kinesthetic means. These are the usual means of remediation; all of them stress the importance of perception. Hours are being spent in the classroom by educators who persist, when the child is 10 or 12 years old, in teaching *to* his deficit area rather than teaching reading around it, through a positive area.

We have agreed that perception is a learned phenomenon. It begins at birth and develops through age six. Equally clear is the fact that there is a difference between peripheral factors and central factors of perception. Most of the differences of understanding about perception lie in what to do about a child with perceptual difficulty after the age of six. Our contention is that, after six years of age, perceptual training is questionable and one should proceed to teach around the deficit, so that years of frustration are not allowed to ensue and the unnecessary expenditures of financial resources allowed to take place. This is exactly where the educator needs to re-think his approach. After a child is beyond age six and is in the early school grades, the teacher's time is largely wasted on efforts to train visual perception. The child's area of deficiency should be identified, and, once this is done, the teacher's time and effort should be given to educational planning of the avenues and directions for teaching the child effectively.

A recent joint statement published by the American Academy of Pediatrics and American Academy of Ophthalmology summarized most appropriately the role of the eyes in learning disabilities. It is a concise statement and is appended at the end of this book, so that the reader who may want to seek further evidence in support of these statements will have access to the appropriate references.

Perceptual training is analogous to a condition called *amblyopia ex anopsia*. In this condition, a child does not develop normal visual acuity of one eye. It is accurate to say that there is no ocular pathology but that the poor visual is due to a central cortical suppression of the visual image of one eye. If this condition is diagnosed before the child is six years of age, proper treatment will restore the vision to normal. However, if it is not diagnosed and treated before this age, then *amblyopia* (poor vision) most often is permanent. Similarly, if a child has a perceptual deficiency that is not diagnosed and treated before the age of six, then perceptual training will probably not develop the skill that is lacking. The child may learn to read but the perceptual deficit may persist even if reading ability increases.

In this chapter, we have sought to explain perception and to emphasize its importance. The tests by which perceptual deficiencies are diagnosed have been given, and an effort has been made to clearly distinguish the peripheral factors of vision from the central factors of perception. As has been indicated, the area of successful treatment for visual-perceptual difficulties lies in the period of reading-readiness, somewhere between birth and the age of six years. It has been well documented that perceptual training after the age of six is of questionable value in the treatment of learning disorders.[70] Such training could be of benefit in the first six years, in the reading-readiness stage, but after this the child makes his own compensations to residual deficits. Thereafter, the time spent in perceptual training could better be spent teaching reading and might well accomplish greater results.

Hearing
and
Auditory
Perception

Auditory

Increasing emphasis is being placed on the development of auditory skills in facilitating the reading process. Johnson and Myklebust (1967)[71] point out that auditory capacity required for reading differs from that required for speaking. Ford (1967) finds audiotory-visual integration to be a significant aspect of reading ability.[72] Of greater significance are those skills that enable a student to sequence auditory stimuli in time. Our traditional concept of hearing has not considered the varieties of separate skills which are now demonstrable as being necessary in the reading process.

Hearing and Auditory Perception

There are many similarities between the visual and auditory apparatus. Just as there are peripheral visual factors, so there are peripheral auditory factors. Similarly, as there are visual-perceptual so there are auditory-perceptual factors in learning disabilities. These perceptual factors involve the central or cerebral mechanisms of learning. Perception is distinguished from sensations and cognition. It occupies an intermediate position between simple peripheral sensations and more complex cognitional behavior.

Hearing is the sensory function that permits an organism to respond to various kinds of acoustic stimuli. The infant responds to the mother's voice, the 6-month-old child responds by turning his head to a source of sounds, a 24-month-old child responds to words and phrases, the 40-month-old child will respond to the details of a sentence, and at the age of five years, the child will normally respond to appropriate learning situations.

A variety of factors can contribute to impaired hearing, such as trauma, infection, genetic factors, and perinatal hypoxia, as a result of mechanical factors attendant on passage through the birth canal.

A differential hearing evaluation allows one to answer five questions: (1) What is the causal picture, (2) is learning involved, (3) how much does the child hear, (4) how does he hear, and (5) what course of treatment is indicated?

During the first month of life as the normal child progresses through stages of reflex sounds and babbling, he depends upon the auditory system for feedback to establish his natural language. Single-word utterances are mastered by the end of the first year of life. The physician who listens to the character of the babble and to the quality of the sound produced may be aware that some children are born with normal hearing which deteriorates during the first year or two of life. All children should utter single words by the first birthday and should say two-word sentences by 24 months of age. Failure to establish single-word utterances, as well as failure to respond adequately to noise in the environment, should alert the examining physician to the possibility of deafness. Routine screening of the hearing ability of the young child requires only simple noise-making toys in a quiet room. Language development begins at birth in the normal child, and any hearing deficit should be handled at this time. The handicap of early childhood deafness is one of the most serious limitations that can befall a child, since it prevents his optimal development and seriously impairs his relationship to the world in which he lives.

The physiologic features of speech involved in peripheral hearing are frequency, rate and intensity. Frequency is the number of vibrations per second produced by a source of sound. Human hearing is concerned with a range of sound waves between 125-8000 cycles per second. Inability to hear consonants in a word is usually characterized by higher frequency loss.

Intensity or loudness is the amount of energy necessary to produce a sound wave and is of importance because the intensity of consonants is weaker compared to that of vowel sounds. Rate is important because it involves the ability to resolve rapidly changing acoustical stimuli into distinctive units of complexity in identifying speech sounds. The more rapidly the speech sounds are produced, the less likely is the ear able to perceive clues of a spoken word. Differences between words are more difficult to hear if the rate is increased.

Measurement of hearing can be obtained by a clinical audiologic appraisal. Two commonly employed kinds of audiologic tests are: (1) those concerned with measurements of acuity in terms of frequency and intensity relative to stimulation by pure tones measured with air-conducted or bone-conducted stimuli, and (2) speech-hearing measurement in terms of minimal acuity level (speech reception threshold) responses that permit generalizations about auditory discrimination relative to various kinds of communicative situations.

The speech-hearing tests are the most important because the child's capacities in interpreting speech are major factors in his ability to learn. Therefore, it is important to know not only how a child hears, but *how much* a child hears. Can the child distinguish and differentiate between sounds that he hears? A child who has difficulty in differentiating between sounds may be a child with a learning disability.

The importance of identifying hearing impairments in children is well-recognized by audiologists, physicians, and educators. All are recognizing the need for early detection of hearing deficits and early diagnosis in order that correctional proceudres can be initiated as early as possible.[73]

If a child cannot hear properly, he cannot understand the instructions given by the teacher. In a group of children studied at the Kennedy Institute in the summer of 1970, it was found that auditory perceptive difficulties were strongly correlated with dyslexia in 54% of the cases.

Auditory perception involves alerting, attention, discrimination, processing, retrieving, sequencing of spoken language, and motor expression of speech. No listening can take place without focusing and attention to the spoken word.

If a child reacts to the wrong signal or if there is too much information for the child to handle, failure might be the result. It is of interest to note how the brain filters messages. There may be numerous voices giving messages, and at a superficial level the brain can absorb many of these stimuli. But if a single message, as an instruction, is received, the brain has power of eliminating extraneous messages and only allows the one to which it is alerted to filter through. Experiments by Cherry are relevant to these conclusions.[74]

Auditory perceptual maturity may not occur until the age of seven. Since only 24% of children have accurate auditory discrimination by the end of the second grade, deficits in this area expose children to the risk of failure.[75]

Perceiving the complex speech code is basic to language. It is not our purpose to discuss or to review the conditions that underlie the perception of speech. This has been extremely well done in a paper by Liberman.[76] For a more elaborate understanding of the analysis of speech, the reader is referred to that article. Our purpose here is to understand what happens between the hearing of the phoneme, the understanding of the speech signals, and speech perception or understanding. It is a result of a complex encoding that makes the sound of speech especially efficient as vehicles for the transmission of auditory information.

For example, a child having difficulty in spelling may write immly for immediately or for the word territory, terote. Normal speech is not as simple as merely the uttering of a few disjointed words, like ship or beet. Words follow one another very rapidly in whole sentences, the listener must associate almost instantaneously in order to follow the meaning and thus gather the thought from the sentence. But just as with visual perception, there is also failure of auditory perception. This type of defect is expressed by the child who says, "I can hear, but I just cannot understand." Interpreting and understanding the teacher often involves more than the acuity of hearing. To illustrate further, a child who writes the following essay on Alexander Hamilton in the fifth grade would normally receive a failing grade because of the spelling. On the other hand, the perceptive and sympathetic teacher should recognize that this child has an auditory imperception and the paper should be marked for its content and not for its spelling.

Example: Written mid-December 1970, Grade Eight

> financlal program full parntyement of war dept incurred by continentel congress. tionpmussa and full payment of state war depts. tremhislbatse of a pound paper yenerrue saf place for publie funds sources of credit finacial agent for S. U. tremnrie- vog. Enactment of higher tarif for revenue and protection levyinsofar excise tax on distilled liquor.

Auditory information is received in groups of letters or syllables called phonemes. A child originally hears the word as a phonemic part, and then gradually builds up the phoneme into a total word. If the child has difficulty in hearing the phoneme, then he could have difficulty in discriminating the entire word. Not only is hearing acuity involved, but also auditory memory. The child has to retain the whole word and discriminate the individual phonemes to contrast the words that he hears. Two examples of tests used for discrimination will be cited. In the Wepman test, the child has to hold the first word which he is given until he hears the second. This involves auditory memory as well as auditory discrimination. These are 40 pairs of words which are sometimes similar and sometimes dissimilar, i.e. both words are repeated and the child is asked to respond "same" or "different." Errors are noted and the results graded according to age. The child who has difficulty in this area might repeat the words *ice cream* as being *nice day*.

Auditory discrimination is the capacity to distinguish between phonemes. Certain conclusions have been summarized by Wepman[77] with reference to auditory discrimination. He concluded that individuals differ in their ability to discriminate sound, that this ability matures until the age of eight years, that slow development of auditory discrimination is correlated with poor pronunciation, and that there is a positive correlation between poor discrimination and poor reading.

There is a group of children who do not seem able to

unravel an auditory message, even though they have normal hearing. These are the children who have an auditory perceptive difficulty, children whose language structure is not sufficient and who begin to encounter academic failure. The diagnosis of aphasia or minimal brain dysfunction may be applied to such children. These are children who cannot follow a series of commands and who are first on the phone at night, calling classmates to ask for the homework assignment. It is not that this happens once or twice, but it is the repeated failure to remember what the teacher has said that makes it unusual. The signals given by the teacher are not carried for a sufficient length of time for such a child to get the message.

In order for a child to compare two or more speech sounds and to make judgments as to their similarity or difference, he must use auditory memory. This is a much more difficult process than visual discrimination and may account for the relatively high frequency of auditory perceptual deficiencies in children with dyslexia.

Tracking is involved when the individual processes information presented orally. Experiments by Foulke (1964), Harley (1966), and Flowers (1964), all referred to in an excellent article by Witkin,[78] suggest that listening comprehension can be improved by training. One interesting observation is that Braille reading occurs at the rate of 90 words per minute, and the average rate of reading of a high school senior is 250 words per minute. The average rate of voice recording for the blind is 175 words per minute. One other interesting observation is that the rate of thought is five times the rate of speech and good listeners utilize this time gap more efficiently than poor listeners.

Information has to be stored, and in some manner information has to be retrieved. This is done by understanding of the word processes. There are certain rules of language acquisition. Some children who have difficulty in learning do not learn simple structured rules. By testing the area of "language processing" we hope to identify weaknesses which would impair learning. Memory, both short-term and long-term, has a part in this process and enhances the ability to learn. Memory tests are available to establish the normal function of this area.

These tests involve digit and sentence repetition. In digit repetition, digits are dictated at a rate of one per second, and then the child is asked to repeat the number of digits which were dictated. Standards have been established which indicate the number of digits which should be remembered when correlated with the age of the child. Sentence repetition, another method of examining for processing, is measured by repeating a sentence which contains a given number of words. The number of words in a sentence are standardized and correlated with age.

Language reception next becomes important for the identification of the source of a child's learning disability. The Peabody Picture Vocabulary Test is a single-word vocabulary test in which four pictures are shown and a single word, describing one of the four pictures, is given. The child is expected then to point to the picture which describes the word. The Durrell is a test for the comprehension of language and consists of short stories which are read to the child. Questions are asked concerning the subject matter read. The results are scored according to grade level.

Closely related to auditory memory is auditory sequencing, which is the recall of sounds in proper time sequence. Sentences are made up of a series of sounds presented in a sequential order. There is some suggestion that impairment in auditory sequential memory is related to reading disabilities, but there is not sufficient observation or research available for a definite statement on the problem.

The subtest of the ITPA for auditory sequencing provides a test for language expression. In this test an envelope, a ball, a button, a piece of chalk, and a block are used. An object is presented and the child tells all that he can about the object. Evaluation is done with reference to the detailed descriptions which the child gives. We are calling on the child to sum up, to articulate, and to categorize the objects which are in front of him. All these factors are important in providing information about auditory perception.

In addition to the peripheral and perceptual aspects of spoken language, there are also the motor aspects of language. If a child of five years has difficulty in speaking, it is possible that he may have had difficulty in the earlier four steps of language development; but if not, there is the possibility of his having a motor disability. A simple example of this difficulty would be the child who is asked to repeat, "the chair is red." The child may attempt to repeat this by saying, "a er e e." A child who has this defect may have had the fault in discrimination, processing, reception, or motor functioning. Varying degrees of disability in any of these areas can make the child a high risk for dyslexia.

Training of defects in these areas can be done. If a child has a hearing loss, then proper amplitude can be obtained by the use of a hearing aid. If he has an auditory perception difficulty, the child can be trained by a series of exercises to improve his auditory perception. A child may be taught to concentrate in conversations with very simple stimuli; or when a child has been taught to remember certain sentences, then perhaps it would be well to teach him to concentrate sufficiently to repeat these sentences when there is some background noise. At the early level at three or four years of age, there are excellent records which can be used to enable the child to identify barnyard sounds, or perhaps to repeat a story to which the child is listening. Each of these simple tasks would help to improve auditory perception.

Children should be studied as they reach school age to determine if their auditory abilities equal their visual abilities. We should not make the mistake of approaching children as if they learned equally well by all systems. Instruction should be individualized to the point of grouping visual learners and auditory learners, at least in the early grades and until the time that the child learns to compensate for any inadequacy in either channel of learning.

Psychiatry and Reading Disabilities

In our present culture, where the ability to accumulate factual information is predominantly through the avenue of reading, the problems of reading disabilities have caused great concern in parent, child, and teacher. However, the question remains as to whether or not psychiatric disturbances can cause learning difficulties or whether or not emotional disorders are a consequence of the child's learning disability.

Actually, both situations are possible. The child who is already overcome by emotional stresses is one who will not learn adequately in the normal school situation. Bryant and Patterson[79] have pointed out that emotional difficulties are almost universal among reading disability cases. They conclude that most children with reading problems feel different, inadequate, stupid, and both frustrated and guilty because of their failures. Conflict and hostility with parents, teachers, and peers often result, along with varied defenses and mechanisms for expressing and controlling these emotions. Thus, in many cases, the emotional problems seem to be a direct result of the failures and conflicts associated with the learning disability.

The psychiatric factors which are important in reading disability fall into two classifications: (1) those arising during the preschool years and (2) those arising after the early school experiences and after entering school. In most cases, the psychiatric factors from the preschool years carry over into the early school years, where new psychiatric factors simply compound the emotional stresses with which the child must try to cope.

Among the factors that are rooted in the preschool years are (1) the child's physical condition, (2) his family and home situations, and (3) his ethnic and/or socioeconomic background.

Regarding the child's physical condition, Denhoff[80] has summarized five conditions at birth which are generally accepted as stress producers: low birth weight, neonatal respiratory stress, high serum bilirubin level, dysmaturity, and anemic diatheses. The signs of these conditions are frequently present during the newborn period or the first year of life, and the symptoms suggesting this condition include tremor, hyperactivity, and seizures. In these preschool years, the confusion and vulnerability to emotional stress of any child with a neurological problem appears only to accentuate emotional problems. The increase in emotional reactivity of individuals following injury to the brain is well known and Bender,[81] among others, has pointed out this emotional vulnerability of children with cerebral malfunctioning. Many observers, including Bakwin and Bakwin,[82] have shown that even a mild degree of brain damage can be the basis for behavioral disturbances, manifested by a low frustration level, impulsiveness, and rapid swings of mood.

One must also consider that anemia and intestinal parasites are some of the physical causes which may bring on malnutrition and lead to emotional stresses. Persistent illness, chronic infections, and other physical handicaps may create emotional stresses that are related to the child's learning readiness. Any difficulty in seeing or hearing is equally related to this and, if not corrected in these preschool years, will complicate and compound the emotionally disturbed child's problems.

Where the family and home-life situation is concerned, there are many possible traumatic events which can create emotional problems in children. The death of a parent, absence of some loved person, or a divorce of the parents are all "loss" situations with traumatic effects that are both immediate and lingering. If there is a divorce situation, the child suffers some of the consternation and warping that a broken home causes.

Kanner cites the case of sisters whose parents were divorced when they were beginning school. For several years the children were shifted back and forth between parents and relatives. When the mother remarried, the stepfather was a cold and impatient perfectionist. The girls often truanted from school. The father lived in New York and one day the girls boarded the train for New York to live with the father. The mother and stepfather were later divorced and the father remarried his original wife. There was no further truancy, and learning problems ceased.[83]

The same is virtually true of a family situation that involves chronic alcoholism or a situation where a parent has a continuing illness. There is no doubt that a child fears for the health of a chronically ill parent and, if this anxiety continues into his school years, he will daydream and be out of contact with reality when the home situation competes for his attention.

His mind wanders to the home situation and he tunes out the classroom teacher.

Almost as traumatic is a constant bickering within the family because of the anxiety that it creates within the child. This is especially true if the child discovers or thinks that he was unwanted and is the center of parental quarrels. When the child fails, the quarrels become more bitter as one or the other of the parents is blamed for the failure. Furthermore, where the home situation is chaotic—for whatever reason—the child is often denied the emotionally stabilizing aspects of love, attention, and discipline that he needs.

Many children from working-class and urban-ghetto homes, in contrast to those from middleclass homes, enter the public school system unprepared for understanding the first-grade curriculum. This is due to a variety of preschool factors that are social, economic, and cultural in nature. The anxieties and emotional problems associated with these children stem from their environment. Hess[84] has found that "the initiative of the mother and her tendency to meet the environment and to enter into interaction with it appear to be important variables in the development of educability in the young child." Put another way, the child from a lower-class, culturally different, or culturally deprived lower-economic environment is apt to react emotionally immediately upon entering public school because of his unpreparedness for a middleclass environment and curriculum. If he is from a different ethnic group, his linguistic and cultural "differentness" promise even more emotional problems and frustrations.

After the child has started school, there are a number of other factors which produce emotional problems. Some are new and some relate to problems from the preschool years. The child who continues to be anemic or chronically ill cannot learn as well as he should. Where family difficulties (alcoholism, divorce, or family quarrels) continue into the school years, the child will daydream and "tune out" the teacher while his mind dwells upon the problems at home. If the child's preschool ethnic, cultural, and socioeconomic background are different, his unfamiliarity with the school setting makes him apprehensive and fearful because there are so many things which he cannot do or understand. If the child is physically immature, or if he has been sheltered at home, his encounters with bullies and militant children in the school environment often create excruciating fears and inhibit his learning.

Three other factors which often occur after the beginning of school are important contributors to psychiatric difficulties: (1) shifting population, (2) sibling rivalry, and (3) aggressive parents. These merit attention in some detail.

One of the greatest problems which the contemporary busing program causes in our current school situation lies in the inexplicable (to the small child) shift from the environment to which he is accustomed. By an artificial change of environment, the child is placed under emotional stress to adjust to the abnormal situation. Although many can do so, some cannot. All experience, to some degree, the emotional stress of adjusting to being bussed from one end of the city to the other, having not only to accommodate to a new school environment, but having to adjust to the new peer relationships, the longer travel time involved, and the often chaotic conditions on the buses themselves.

There is no doubt that the busing of children to schools beyond their normal environment has produced unnecessary anxieties in all children. Belligerency and open militancy forbid an atmosphere conducive to study. The emotional disadvantages of such a program far outweigh any advantages of equal educational opportunity. There were other ways tò achieve this opportunity, and failure to recognize these methods has produced irreparable harm and has increased the educational stress of some children. Not only is local busing educationally upsetting insofar as it creates stresses by changing the child's environment, but the traditional mobility of Americans contributes to frequent shifts of children from one section of the country to another. One in four American families move each year. A first-grader or second-grader who is forced to go from one region to another because of family or economic reasons, military transfer of his family, or for any other of the myriad of reasons, is going to have difficulty in adjusting to the different teaching methods, differences in dialects, and even differences in curriculum. Frequently, the child is uprooted in midyear. There may be difficulty in the family's settling down again, and the child may even visit three or four schools in a year's time. This child will most certainly have difficulty.

A child learns his own sectional dialect and feels comfortable with it. If he is transported to another section where a different dialect is spoken, he becomes somewhat insecure and has difficulty. In learning to read, the emotional stress and confusion over different dialects (whether cultural or geographic) will cause a child to be confused as to the true meaning of spoken language and the written language. To avoid these psychiatric problems, therefore, it is better to have a stable environment in which the child feels comfortable and secure.

Another major cause of consternation and failure in children is the factor of sibling rivalry. The fact that Mary has performed well in school does not mean that her brother John, following her, will do as well. Both teachers and parents often place extreme and unwarranted pressure upon the second child, when they are actually dealing with two individual children. One child may have a greater capacity for learning than the other, or may learn at a faster rate than the other, or may be better motivated to learn, or may even have a different interest than the other sibling. The sibling rivalry always sets up unfair and invidious comparisons and makes learning far more difficult for the younger child and occasionally even for the older child.

Somewhat related to this is the "aggressive parent situation." The rule, "Expectancy, when not correlated with observed behavior, means that the child is headed for trouble," is meaningful here.

Not until a child is of school age does the parent see the child in real competition with other children. So far the child has been in competition only at play, and there have been no standards of measure by which he could be compared. Perhaps another child did speak a little earlier or is a little keener at certain things, but the parent can always rationalize an apparent inadequacy by saying, "Johnny walked earlier," or perhaps find another area in which there is a halo effect. He never sees the whole picture, and it is not until the child enters school that he finds established standards against which he can be compared with others his own age. When this happens, the very desire of the parent to see his child excel may often lie at the heart of that child's inability to perform as well as other children. Such strong desire for achievement is usually accompanied by tensions and anxieties which can easily affect the child's learning process.

When parents expect more of a child than he is capable of performing, trouble is in the offing. Such a child, unable to meet expectations, will accumulate emotional problems, including resentment, hostility, and guilt. He will carry a constant burden of guilt because he cannot measure up to the older brother or sister or to the ideal in the parental mind. Often, with aggressive parents, the child is expected to perform at some ideal level merely to satisy the parental ego. Such expectations, unrealizable by the child, produce hostility and a resentment toward the pattern-figure, i.e. the older brother or sister and the parents themselves.

Regarding other factors, a very interesting study, conducted at Duke University, was published by Spielberger,[85] who had worked with students divided into two groups: the high-anxiety student and the low-anxiety student. He found that the failures in the high-anxiety group amounted to 20.2%, while the failure rate in the low-anxiety group was only 5.8%. Diethelm[86] found that, in psychiatric institutions, the children were unable to perform certain tests adequately when the tension was increased in the hosptial atmosphere. Thus, there is ample support for the conclusion that apprehension and tension are causative factors in failure.

This may be illustrated from individual cases. The author has seen many children who were referred to him because they had failed the Benton Visual Memory Test in the schools. In retesting them, the anxiety factor became visible. For example, there was a child who performed normally when retested in the examiner's office. Yet he had been diagnosed by school authorities as brain-damaged and suffering from perceptual loss. Unable to reconcile these findings, the child was tested again, this time in the presence of his mother, who manifested extreme aggressiveness. This time, the child failed completely on all aspects of the test. However, as soon as the child was alone and the test was again given without any parental pressure, the child performed the test successfully.

Surely these illustrations of the relationship between failure and anxiety should lead us to conclude that a child should be measured by his own abilities. Certainly one should not constantly elevate tensions by comparing a child with the sibling or parent who might have achieved a high measure of success in school. Aggression that demands superior performance at some level demanded by the parent's ego only creates in a child the most crippling of anxieties. It is as unrealistic and damaging to a child to demand performance beyond his capabilities as it is to frankly demand that he be another Einstein or Pasteur. People are different and, even in the same family, children should be evaluated as separate persons. The overambitious and aggressive parent causes only confusion, apprehension, and failure in the child confronted by some ideal model or sibling rival.

The child who is beset with problems of this nature will react to his failures in several ways. In fact, there is a certain progression, or series of steps of reaction, which may be summarized as follows: (1) a "couldn't care less" attitude, (2) a paranoid attitude toward his teacher, (3) marked feelings of inferiority, and (4) a tendency toward emotional blocking and frank aggressiveness toward others.

If a child is failing and receiving no understanding, the child will normally reject the learning situation. He may say, "I just couldn't care less," or "I just do not want to learn," or "It is not important." Or, he may not verbalize any of these but say them through his actions of indifference and rejection of the learning process.

If the matter of his failure is pursued by his parents or the teacher, there follows the development of a paranoid reaction toward the teacher. The unresolved problem of failure is transferred to the teacher and the child complains, "The teacher just picks on me," or "The teacher doesn't like me," or "I can't learn the way she teaches." Thus, for a number of reasons, the teacher becomes the focus of the child's failure.

When failure cannot be successfully transferred to the teacher, feelings of marked inferiority often follow. If the child continues to fail and the effort to blame the teacher has failed, then the child begins to accept the idea that he is at fault. He has been told repeatedly that he is stupid and lazy and that he just does not have it in him to perform satisfactorily. There is a loss of self-esteem and ego status, and the subsequent step is emotional blocking and frank aggressiveness.

In this final stage, the child has to be forced to go to school. He tunes out the teacher completely, daydreams, and tries to dismiss the whole problem from his mind, thus emotionally blocking out any possible learning experience. If pressed to perform, the child reacts with undisguised hostility and aggressiveness. He will try to destroy the learning situation which causes his emotional turmoil. At this point, he may disrupt classes, bullying other students, smashing classroom displays and furnishings, and terrorizing the school. When these hostile and destructive tendencies are frustrated, he plays "hooky," becomes a school dropout, and, frequently, a delinquent.

In some cases, such children will actually try to burn the school. Children who have reached this point of psychiatric disturbance are no longer just a school problem but a problem for society itself. This is supported by Harrower's[87] finding that 75% of juvenile delinquents in the New York area had some form of reading disability, and by Judge James H. Lincoln's[88] statement that "Most chronic delinquents read at three or four grades below their average grade placement. They're the lowest achievers among drop-outs. They account for 90 percent of the severe behavior problems in this country." What Judge Lincoln of Detroit, the new president of the National Council of Juvenile Court Judges, is emphasizing is that the burning of schools and other severe behavioral problems often have their beginnings back in the home and in the early classroom situation.

In studying children with reading problems, psychiatric researchers have found almost all of them to be difficult, restless, and upset. In a study reported by Ingram and Reid,[89] it was found that, among 78 cases, 20% came from broken homes, another 20% were from homes with intermittent parental separation, and 25% had parents who were in need of, or receiving, psychiatric treatment. Fabian[90] found, among 20 cases, persisting traits of immaturity in the children and mild-to-severe signs of psychopathology in their families. Blanchard[91] in still another study concluded that failure to learn to read is a consequence of negative attitudes toward parents being transferred to teachers.

Missildine[92] has reported a study of 30 cases of children having reading problems. They were all children of normal intelligence, selected at random from the files of a reading clinic. His report reads in part:

> Twenty of these thirty children came from homes where the mothers, if not overtly hostile, were of a coercive, perfectionistic nature. Four of the children felt that a small sibling at home was getting the maternal attention which they coveted. Two others were indulged until they entered school and then either neglected or frankly rejected. One child's emotional troubles were largely on the basis of geography: she wanted to be back in her home in Tennessee. The loyalties of another child were divided between two families, both of which contained emotionally disturbing elements. Finally, two of our children were overprotected. One of these lacked sufficient motivation to learn to read, while the other reflected his father's nervousness and his mother's hyperthyroidism.
>
> All of these children, with at most one or two exceptions, had this in common: they harbored a serious disturbance in connection with some member or members of their families. Some assumed a restless, indifferent, happy-go-lucky pose in re-

acting to this disturbance. Others felt crushed, unhappy and inadequate.

Whether the psychiatric problem is the cause of reading difficulty or a result of it, the introverted child may become more introverted, and the extroverted child may react in a belligerent manner which can end in serious problems of major delinquency. One thing that is manifested by both types is an utter dislike for reading, and the very sight of a book may cause the feeling of resentment. Breaking down these antagonisms is a problem for the child, and the parent may often play an important role.

Alarmed, puzzled, and defensive when their child does not do well in reading, some parents try to prove both to themselves and to their neighbors that their child is not handicapped. This apprehension is reflected in the emotional state of the child and makes reading even more difficult. A parent may sit very calmly with a child to teach him that *these, them,* and *those* are three separate words. He may patiently explain the spelling of the words; even spell them out on paper and have the child spell them after him. But the child will confuse the words time and time again. Soon the parent becomes more and more frustrated until in anger he explodes, slapping the child, or shoving the table away and calling the child "stupid" or "lazy." The child is confused by all this. He may be trying very hard to do the right thing, but he simply does not have the tools to work with. The result may be that the child begins to resent the parent. If the parent sits down again with him, even in a calm moment, the child no longer trusts his parent and fears an explosion is imminent. It has now become impossible for the parent to give any assistance at all.

The reading environment at home is most important, and an active cooperation between teacher, parent, and student is needed to help in these cases. Perhaps there is another member of the class who can help the child who is having difficulty. Perhaps a neighbor will come in to assist the child. The neighbor is far less likely to become emotionally involved than is the parent, and may be able to lend a great deal of assistance.

I cannot stress too much the importance of a parent understanding the limitations of his child, treating him as an individual, and trying not to push him beyond his capabilities. Before a child reaches school age the parent should be aware of the child's reading readiness, and be prepared for problems should they arise.

So many times parents have said, "I just can't help Johnny any more. He doesn't seem to understand. He doesn't seem to want to learn. I try to help him, but he complains. He dawdles at his work, and I just don't know where to turn next. My patience is at an end." Msot teacher do not seem to be making an effort to understand the parental problem. Only at specially motivated reading clinics will the whole problem be understood, and there are too few of these at the present time. Usually it is the pediatrician who comes in contact with these cases first, and whether or not he is familiar with the problem may make a great difference to the child's future reading abilities.

The child who cannot read may appear in the pediatrician's office in a variety of symptomatic guises. Only rarely do the parents admit to the doctor that they are perplexed over their child's inability to read. Most commonly the chief complaint is poor school progress, with reading difficulty mentioned only incidentally or not at all as a specific concern. The child who is intelligent is often able to disguise his inability to read by making use of auditory learning to memorize passages in his primer, which he appears to read as he actually repeats them by rote. As the nonreader ascends through the primary grades, his problem multiplies because most other subject matter requires reading. So, it becomes impossible for him to solve the arithmetic or social studies problems, simply because he cannot read the examination question itself, even though he may have the other necessary skills. The impression is one of general academic failure. He is likely to be considered as mentally retarded or as a lazy child, with the formula "he could if he would."

Much has been said about the poor reader in our school system. However, the child with a high intellectual capacity and who performs in an inadequate manner is of considerable concern. This is the child who has an IQ of 125 but reads below grade level. This student in high school studies an unreasonable number of hours, but barely passes his subjects. He may attend college because his high IQ has enabled him to compensate for his difficulty in reading. At the college level he may rebel or never reach his true potential. This tragic loss may be the result of an unrecognized reading disability. This could account for the varying degrees of success as perhaps demonstrated by the Lee Harvey Oswald or the college graduate who "just never found himself."

Such an accusation must be devastating to the child who is confused by his inability to learn in spite of his honest efforts to do so. Failure by teacher, parent, and physician to recognize the key problem may have serious results. Frustrated by his inability to learn, bored by class exercises he cannot follow, coerced by parents and teachers to do what he cannot, the nonreader has both the inner turmoil and the lack of constructive outlet to become a major problem at home and at school. The only way serious psychological consequences can be averted is by recognition as a reading disability by parent, teacher, and physician, of a condition usually presenting itself either as a problem of scholastic failure or as a behavior disorder. Many studies of juvenile delinquents have stressed the high proportion of nonreaders that are to be found among them. It is entirely possible that inability to read can contribute significantly to the rebellious attitude toward society, as the youngster, frustrated by his repeated academic failure, seeks his place in the sun through channels disapproved by adults.

To disentangle cause and effect is a massive task which, up to now, has not been adequately undertaken. It is nevertheless understood that the reading problem itself provides a major barrier to successful rehabilitation of these youngsters within the framework of public schooling unless special attention is directed toward remedial reading measures.

It is not a difficult matter for a physician to identify a retarded reader. No more than 5 minutes are required for giving a simple clinical reading test that is available. Other, carefully standardized tests, like the Gray Oral Reading Paragraphs and the Gates Primary Reading Tests, permit a more precise evaluation of reading performance. Pediatricians are encouraged to make such tests when confronted with academic failures or behavior problems, because the key to successful treatment lies in early recognition of the problem. The longer the difficulty persists, the greater is the degree of general academic retardation and the more distressing the whole train of emotional consequences. Success with therapy may be said to vary inversely with the length of time the problem has persisted.

The child who has a major psychiatric problem will need psychiatric treatment concurrently with his remedial reading therapy, or may even need psychotherapy for an initial period in order to prepare him to accept reading help.

The family is best advised to cease pushing the child, to avoid home teaching, which usually proves frustrating to parents as well as to the child, and to concentrate on building a better relationship with him by developing his self-confidence about things he *can* do well. At the same time, specific problems in family-child relations require understanding, an opportunity for expression and sympathetic guidance from the physician.

There is reason to believe that methods for the early detection and rehabilitation of children with reading disorders may make a significant contribution to the problem of juvenile delinquency. The high rate of reading disability among delinquents suggests, at least, that some of their poor motivation and their antisocial behavior may be caused partly by the repeated experience of frustration and failure they experience from their reading difficulty.

It is well recognized that males exceed females in reading disabilities by a frequency that varies from 3:1 to 10:1. The greater male incidence can be explained by the following possibilities:

(1) Greater female maturity at the age of six.

(2) Greater incidence of cerebral trauma accompanying retinal and cerebral hemorrhages.

(3) Greater motivation of females in the learning situation.

(4) Secondary emotional conflict in the male associated with (1)–(3) above.

Having established that children do in fact react poorly to the learning situation because of factors that exist prior to and which develop after the beginning of school, and after describing the ways in which a child reacts to failure, now we ought to establish some goals for the psychiatric care of such children. These goals are best described by Kanner[93] as the "Five R's" of psychotherapy: (1) relieve, (2) relate, (3) release, (4) relearn, and (5) relax.

First of all, the family situation must be *relieved*. The home environment is basic and the emotional pressures there must be dealt with. It is in this situation that the social worker with an undertanding of psychiatric factors as they relate to reading can be of extreme value in contributing to an understanding of the family situation. A visit to the home, a review of the child's work habits, a look at the contributions of father and mother to motivating the child, and the relationship of siblings to each other can do more to provide background material than many visits to the psychiatrist's office. This effort by the psychiatric social worker is poorly understood and structured, but understanding of the social worker's contributions will go a long way toward alleviating the learning problem.

Whether the problem is alcohol, parental incompatibility, divorce, death or chronic illness, or simply sibling rivalry and overly ambitious parents, the family situation must be relieved. Both public and private agencies can be called in for help in some of these cases. Often, the family needs only reassurance that the child is not stupid or lazy or brain-damaged and an explanation of what the reasonable expectancy of performance of the child might be. Group conferences with the parents, even with the whole family, may be helpful in taking the crippling burden of emotional stresses from the child.

Secondly, one should *relate* to the child. One should relate to the child and let him know that he has a friend. As a friend, try to establish some rapport with the child and let him feel that someone is sympathetically concerned about the problem with which he is struggling. Above all, one should try to encourage the child into those techniques and areas of learning in which he is proficient and through which he can expect some successes.

Thirdly, help him *release* his emotions. One should encourage the child to express how he feels about the learning situation. Let him release his emotions of frustration and resentment toward the teacher, his parents, or his fellow students. The child who has these pent-up feelings must be able to talk with someone. Otherwise, there is no real way for him to get a good assessment of who he is and what his difficulties are.

Fourth, we need to help him *relearn* his role in life and in society. Perhaps he is not going to be an academically oriented student. If a child has an IQ of only 80, we want to give him realistic goals. If one child's IQ is 100 and his brother's is 140, we should differentiate the goals of the two boys and set up different levels of expectation for both children and for the parents. Certainly there are aspects of talent and motivation in every child which can be related to goals which he can achieve and thus become proficient. If he does not perform at an expectancy rate which is equivalent to his brother's or his parents' expectations, then frankly reestablish what his expectations are.

One should at least let a child feel success in whatever area he wants to adopt as his role in life. He may not be destined for superiority in the traditional academic world. Other goals are worthy; they can be established, and should be accepted by the parents. Teachers also ought to recognize that a child who does not work well in the routine academic subjects need not be a failure. He may pursue the fine arts, music, painting, or some vocational work. A child can become just as successful an individual if he works with his hands in the mechanical world as in the academic world. He will certainly be happier in fulfilling his role in life if he can find an area in which he is proficient and where his work is personally satisfying.

Finally, the fifth "R" means *relax*. It means that *everyone* involved must relax. With his emotional tensions eased, the child can attack his learning problems better. With the family and parental pressures having given way to a better understanding of the problem, there is an opportunity to establish more realistic expectations. The teacher is better able to guide and instruct the child if these expectations are realistic. The physician, the psychologist, the psychiatrist, or other paramedical personnel can act as a relaxed go-between for all, so that everyone can feel that a common goal has been acquired, to which the child can relate in a realistic way and toward which he can progress satisfactorily. After all, the principle goal of any psychotherapy or—in a broader sense, of all mental hygiene—is an effort to attempt to help a person to retain or regain his optimal condition of comfort and smoothness of functioning. One cannot exist without the other. Where there is no smoothness of functioning, there is no comfort, and where there is no comfort, no smoothness of functioning can be expected.

The Role of Dominance

Observation has shown that, while lobsters and crabs prefer to use the right claw and the great majority of rats have a preference for the right paw,[94] in general animals are nearly always ambidextrous and show no preference for a particular paw or foot.* The human species was originally ambidextrous, too. A study of cave paintings and tools employed by Stone Age man has revealed that there were about as many right-handed as left-handed individuals among our remote ancestors.

Right-hand dominance suddenly appeared in the Bronze Age. The reason for this is unknown, but there is a "weapon theory" that speculates that the right-handed individuals of the hunter-warrior Stone Age period survived because they carried their weapons in the right hand and protected their hearts by means of a shield. In any event, we know that the priority of the right hand was established in man during the more settled and agricultural Bronze Age because their scythes were designed for wielding by right-handed individuals.

The emergence of laterality in mankind, with dominance of

---

*Incidentally this preference can be annulled by drugs, such as acetylcholine, or by removal of part of the motor area of the *left* (opposite) side of the brain.

one side of the body, usually the right eye, the right hand and foot, under the control of the left cerebral hemisphere, is a subject that has been fully explored and has a social significance that is often overlooked. In discussing facial asymetry, for example, Hutter[2] suggested that the right half of the face is imprinted with the individual's attitudes toward life, while the left half expresses those extra aspects and the hidden traits of temperament which are governed by the individual's subconscious process. It has been said that each of us is divided into a "left person" which is gayer and more extrovertive, and a "right person" which is more introvertive and meditative.

Texts taken from the Bible and from the *Iliad*[95] show that the distinction between right-handed and left-handed men has aroused the curiosity of researchers from the earliest times. Human beings tend to fall into these two categories, but right-handed and left-handed persons are not simply mirror images of each other. The larger group is composed of right-handed individuals whose language centers are situated in the left hemisphere of the brain. Dominance of the right foot is usually associated with dominance of the right hand. The smaller group consists of left-handed persons whose language centers are usually located in the right hemisphere of the brain.

Many investigators have described in detail the successive bilateral and unilateral stages through which the growing child passes before the right-handed or left-handed tendency becomes permanently established. However, the precise age at which this handedness is settled is subject to great individual variation. There are a number of time intervals given by various writers. One feels that there is established a right-handed tendency in the eighth month of life. Another places this at the age of five years. Still others feel that the age of one year is the time when the differentiation of an active hand and a passive hand begins. At 18 months the two hands parallel each other in their movement, but after two years the passive hand becomes increasingly subordinate. This happens to coincide with language development. Handedness and language develop earlier in girls than in boys. One would expect this because of the greater maturity of females at this period of life. One can conclude that, generally, hand differentiation begins in the child at about nine months and is virtually complete by two years of age.

Today, dominance of the left hand occurs in approximately 5%–10% of the population of the United States. Left-hand dominance is twice as common in boys than in girls, and it is twice again as common in imbeciles. Evidences for the pathological aspect of left-handedness is provided by Gordon,[96] who studied 219 pairs of twins and showed that, when one twin is right-handed and the other is left-handed, the left-handed twin often shows some evidence of mental abnormality. Other investigators have found a greater frequency of left-handedness among retarded children. Left-handedness is frequently associated with perinatal distress and also with abnormal EEG findings. Gordon found that in regular schools 7.2% of the children were left-handers, while in schools for handicapped children the incidence of left-handedness soared to 18.2%.

Handedness results not only from genetic possibilities but from the relationship of genetic possibilities with parental attitudes. These parental attitudes toward handedness result from their social, vocational, economic, and educational experiences. However, pure left-handedness is extremely rare. In a study by Subirana,[97] out of 316 children only one case was found. The fact is that pure right-handedness is also rare. In this same group of 316 children, only 25 pure right-handers were found.

Right-handed individuals tend to write from left to right, while some left-handed persons tend to mirror-write from right to left. The Phoenicians wrote from right to left, as did their Semitic successors. The Greeks often had to reverse the orientation of their left-to-right script. This actually produced a period of writing lines in alternate directions, called Boustrophedon, which is after the pattern of ox-plowing. However, by the fourth century B.C., both Greek and Roman writings were uniformly right-handed (dextrad).

The relationship between handedness and eyedness is very interesting. Man is primarily and innately right-eyed or left-eyed and only secondarily right- or left-handed. Ninety percent of individuals are right-handed but only two-thirds of them are both right-handed and right-eyed. Similarly, while only about 7% are left-handed, left-eyedness occurs in 30% of individuals. Actually, therefore, one-third of individuals have a mixed dominance of hand and eye. In Subirana's[98] study of 316 children, he found in 143 a lack of agreement in eye and hand preference. Learning disabilities associated with a conflict of handedness and footedness were found in 16% of these children. This discordant lateralization may be compensated for by the child's subsequent maturation.

Most individuals have a preference for monocular sighting and this preference is established earlier than hand preference. The master eye is usually the one with preferential visual acuity. In some persons, the optically weaker eye may be preferred for sighting. In dominance, eyedness is a more significant finding because the person is not aware of his preferred eye and environmentally is not encouraged to change this dominance.

Artists are usually right-handed and, when painting in the daylight, they tend to position the window on their left side. The model is placed somewhat to the painter's left and nearer to the window, which illuminates the right side of the model's face. The model's right eye, or the master eye, looks directly at the artist and the left eye is allowed the freedom of a little divergence. When an artist paints a self-portrait, the right side of the face is illuminated but the left eye appears to be the master eye.

An associated dominance of the right eye was first noted in 1883 by Lombroso. This eye preference probably underlies foot and hand dominance, since the eye controls the hand. All three, the foot, the hand, and the eye, were related to the opposite side of the cerebral hemisphere. Of course, there is no absolute separation of left and right, and many interweaving grades of ambidexterity exist. The laterality of the brain is something that is genetically induced, generally as a recessive trait.

Another aspect of this hemicerebral dominance is the dominance of the field of vision that corresponds to the master eye. There is a greater ease in directional scanning toward that field of vision. Persons with right-hand dominance find the right-hand side of the page easier to register and the eyes sweep more easily to that side than away from it.

The concept of hemispheric cerebral localization is found in the Hippocratic writings about 400 B. C., which made the observation that a wound in the left temple produces a spasm in the oposite side of the body. The Frenchman Pourfour du Petit demonstrated this fact experimentally in animals in 1710 and Morgagni, the great Italian anatomist, established it for man in the same century.

The concept of cerebral hemispheric dominance is only 100 years old. It arose out of Broca's observation in 1861 of the association between aphasia and lesions of the left frontal lobe. Broca' observations were made with extreme caution and it was not until 1865 that Broca finally advanced the idea that aphasia was specifically related to disease of the left hemisphere.

At this same time, there was postulated a relationship between handedness and hemispheric cerebral dominance for language. There was some question as to what the role of the minor, or nondominant, hemisphere might be. There were some who thought that it might be a silent partner, participating in a supportive way in normal speech and capable of assuming the other function of speech mediation if the dominant hemisphere were put out of action by injury or disease. Others felt that the lesser hemisphere was the center for musical language. Still others[99] have felt that the lesser cerebral hemisphere embraces a much broader range of activity.

The two hemispheres (halves) of the brain, anatomically, are jointed together at several points. One is at the common stem that descends from the brain into the spinal cord, otherwise known as the medulla oblongata. Two other areas of possible junction are at the optic chiasm and at the cerebellum. A fourth connection, known as the great cerebral commissure, is made by means of the corpus callosum, and in this area much experimentation is taking place.

A task is learned in one of two ways: (1) by one hemisphere transmitting the information to the other at the time the initial learning takes place, or (2) by supplying it on demand later. In the first instance, intercommunication by way of the corpus callosum at the time of the learning results in the formation of a double set of memory traces, one in each half of the brain. In the second case, a set of engrams is established only in the directly trained half, but this information is available to the other hemisphere, when it is required, by way of the corpus callosum.

It was thought at one time that the corpus callosum was crucial for the proper performance of the brain functions.

However, it has been noted recently that the corpus callosum can be cut in humans and in animals without any loss of function. In fact, the two halves of the brain can learn diametrically opposite solutions to the same experimental problem.

R. E. Myers[100] in 1962 reported that a sectioning of the corpus callosum, a procedure that prevents communication between the two halves of the brain, could demonstrate the interaction between the two hemispheres. If a normal animal is trained to do a trick with one paw, it can be shown that he will also know this trick with the other paw. After the trick has been learned with the left paw, even a sectioning of the corpus callosum will not prevent its being known by the right paw. If, however, the section is made before the trick is learned by one paw, it has to be learned all over again by the other. Evidentally, in the normal animal, what is learned by one brain hemisphere is transmitted by the corpus callosum to the other hemisphere and retained there as a learned pattern useful also for the other hemisphere.

R. W. Sperry,[101] professor of psychobiology at the California Institute of Technology, reported experiments on cats, monkeys, and chimps in which they were subjected to surgical operations that cut through the corpus callosum, so that the two brain hemispheres were completely separated. Each half of the split brain was then tested in a series of experiments to determine perception of learning, visual and tactile discrimination, and motor responses. These animals showed little disturbance resulting from the operation, but the tests indicated a complete loss of normal carry-over of learning from one brain hemisphere to the other. If an animal was taught a task and then the corpus callosum was sectioned, thereby dividing the two parts of the brain, the animal could perform the task after section. However, if the task was taught after a section of the corpus callosum, and then one part of the brain was removed, the animal could not perform the task, since there was no sharing of the two hemispheres.

Sperry offers the opinion that in man, where one hemisphere is nearly always dominant, the single engram system tends to prevail, particularly in all memory related to language. Sperry feels that in the human brain, specialization of language takes place in the separation of functions of the two hemispheres. Language is the task of the dominant hemisphere and lesser tasks are taken over by the other hemisphere. The non-dominant hemisphere, however, apparently possesses the potential to take over the normal function of the naturally dominant hemisphere if the latter is incapacitated by injury in the young child. If contradictory tasks were taught to the separate brain hemispheres of the monkey, the results indicated that one hemisphere or the other would always take command. Sperry wondered whether or not the normally intact brain is sometimes subject to conflicts that are attributable to the brain's double structure.

Proof of the fact that these experiments in memory do not apply absolutely to man is suggested by the evidence that patients who are operated on for intractable epilepsy by cutting the commissures will have their epilepsy cured but suffer no disability in memory. Another notable exception is that, if the corpus callosum fails to develop because of some congenital anomaly, centers for language and other functions may develop in compensation on both sides of the brain. Normally, however, training transfers from one side of the brain to the other, but when the corpus callosum is impaired the subsequent training of one does not help the other side.

The corpus callosum experiments show that (1) both sides of the brain share learning engrams in the cat; (2) the monkey brain sometimes uses the double engram system but, under certain conditions, training may lay down engrams in only one of its hemispheres; and (3) in man, where the one hemisphere is nearly always dominant, the single engram system tends to prevail, particularly in all memory functions related to language.

It is generally recognized that when a right-handed person has a cerebral vascular accident or stroke affecting the left hemisphere, he develops a paralysis on the right side of the body. Conversely, if it affects the right hemisphere, he suffers from a paralysis on the left side. Injuries of the temporal parietal area on the right side produce a disturbance of spatial perception, loss of awareness of body scheme, and loss of spatial relationships. A corresponding injury on the left side has the effect of producing the most severe disruption of language and its associated thought processes. This raises the possibility that the right hemisphere assumes a dominant role for spatial relationships and the left hemisphere a dominant role for temporal relationships. If one assumes that for the language function the temporal relationships are most crucial, then it is logical for the language function to be developed in the left hemisphere of the brain.

A change in dominance can be brought about under two pathological conditions: (1) injury to the dominant hand or (2) injury to the dominant hemisphere of the brain. For example, a child who was right-handed had his right hand amputated at the age of six. He became pathologically left-handed. Twenty-one years later this child, now an adult, developed a tumor in the right hemisphere which required removal of this right hemisphere. The patient lost the power of speech (aphasia) because the dominance had shifted to the right hemisphere. This is one example of a shift in dominance as a result of a peripheral defect, occurring only after an early change in peripheral stimulation and only after 21 years of training.

Insofar as injuries to the dominant brain hemisphere itself are concerned, there was a study of 522 patients upon whom brain operations were performed for treatment of focal cerebral seizures. Among these cases were some who developed aphasia after surgery on the left hemisphere, even though it had been previously damaged by the original disease or injury. Thus, even though there was injury to the left cerebral cortex, the left cortex retained the power of speech until the operation knocked it out. This demonstrates how difficult it is to change dominance.

Penfield and Roberts[102] summarized a study of a group of individuals who experienced language impairment after brain operations. Of the 157 right-handed persons who had operations on the left side of the brain, 78% developed aphasia. Of those who were left-handed and who also had operations on the left side of the brain, 72% became aphasic. Thus, even of the left-handed individuals in this study a large majority still had the center for language on the left side of the brain.

In the patient who has left-hemisphere dominance, language is found in this area in a ratio of 97% to 3%. This is not true however, in left-handed individuals. In this group, lesions in the right hemisphere in the left-handed individual need not produce an aphasia or language disability in more than 59%

of the cases. And if there is a right-hemisphere involvement, only 41% will be left-handed. Thus, left-hemisphere dominance is more likely to be consistent. But right-hemisphere dominance is not consistent with aphasia when surgery is done to the respective hemisphere.

Rasmussen[103] found that patients in whom left-handedness was due to early brain damage were more likely to have speech in the right hemisphere. But 22% still had speech facility in the left side. Penfield felt that the speech capability remains on the left side, even in left-handed patients. The fact that a patient is left-handed indicates that unilateral dominance is less strongly developed and speech often tends to be bilaterally represented. When there is clinical evidence of brain injury on the left side at birth, speech was found to be located on the right side of the brain in 66% of cases and on the left side in 33% of cases.

The significance of these findings is that the dominant brain hemisphere for language is most often the left one. Even in individuals who are left-handed by ordinary standards, the left hemisphere is still very likely to be dominant for the language function. An exception to this lies in the fact that an injury to the dominant hemisphere incurred in childhood can be compensated for by a shift of dominance to the opposite hemisphere. Thus, although the language function in most persons is subserved primarily by the left hemisphere, the right hemisphere has the capability for this task if the task is forced upon it. This transfer of dominance rarely occurs in adults and is usually successful only in children under the age of eight years.

Hugo Liepmann, a German neurologist, was the first to define apraxia as a distinctive category of behavioral deficits shown by patients with cerebral disease. Apraxia is the inability to perform a skilled act or series of movements. There are a number of types of this disability, and one is called "ideomotor apraxia." This is the inability to perform familiar acts on verbal command or by imitation, such as making a fist or saluting or waving good-by. Liepmann felt that apraxia resulted from a lesion of the left dominant hemisphere. In the 1920's Gerstmann described an unusual deficit associated with lesions of the major hemisphere. The parts of this syndrome, known as Gerstmann's syndrome, were (1) finger agnosia, or the inability to identify fingers on tactile stimulaton, (2) loss of ability to discriminate left and right side of the body, (3) loss of ability to write (agraphia), and (4) the loss of the ability to do mathematics (acalcalia).

The question has been raised as to whether the non-dominant hemisphere does not have some distinctive function with respect to behavior. British and French neurologists have called attention to the fact that deficits in the right nondominant hemisphere have produced impairment in visual space perception, constructional apraxia, apraxia for dressing, and inattention to one-half of the visual field. Therefore, this group of symptoms from both the major and the minor hemispheres all produce the possibility of those symptoms frequently found in children who have dyslexia. In other words, dyslexia can occur from a dysfunction in either the major or minor hemisphere.

Furthermore, there is a question as to the role of the right hemisphere in right-handed individuals—that is, of the lesser hemisphere. Critchley[104] has suggested that the right hemisphere plays a significant role in mediating higher-level language performances of the right-handed individuals, with the left hemisphere subserving more basic language processes. Eisenson in 1962 had shown that patients with right-hemisphere lesions perform more poorly than a normal subject on tests of vocabulary recognition and sentence construction. In a schematic way there are certain conclusions that can be drawn from patients with minor or nondominant hemispheric lesions: (1) They show a greater impairment in spatial perception and memory as expressed by difficulty in following or remembering routes, or by an inability to locate places on a map. (2) There is impairment in visuoconstructive activity, the so-called constructional apraxia—for example, the inability to copy or to draw a design of one's house. (3) Defects exist in visual perception and memory for nonverbal material, such as scenic representations, faces, or abstract figures. (4) Impairment in certain aspects of auditory perception and memory is more frequently encountered in patients with right-hemispheric lesions. (5) There is also a motor impersistence which consists of the inability of the patient to sustain a movement that he has been able to initiate on verbal command, such as keeping his eyes closed or keeping the tongue protruding. Each of these five points are found more frequently in patients with minor-hemispheric lesions.

Increasing evidence has been accumulated by some professionals for the assumed correlation of certain disorders in children's language development with delayed or incomplete establishment of preferential laterality. However, Brain[105] and Subirana[106] both state that poor dominance or ill-defined laterality is not a cause of language difficulty; rather, it is a concomitant symptom reflected on a parallel level. The basic deviation of brain function is responsible for both language and laterality disorders. In other words, if there is cerebral immaturity, there will be disorders of laterality and of learning.

The question of the confusion as to the role of dominance—whether it is cause or effect—was first raised by Orton[107] in 1937. The view presented by Orton was that many of the delays and defects in the development of the language function may result from a deviation in the process of establishing unilateral brain superiority. This concept of hemispheric dominance was a sensation among educators and Orton's views were widely circulated. Left-handedness in cases of dyslexia was frequent, and some disorder of dominance was a convenient explanation. But the answer is not so simple. There are many exhaustive tests for eye, hand, foot, and ear dominance. In a study of 100 achieving students, there would be no statistically significant difference between the dominance of those who are achieving poorly and those who are successful. The theory that individuals with severe reading disability have poorly lateralized dominance may be because 20% of these children may have some form of brain dysfunction, which may lead to poor lateralization and poor learning. In these cases, the poor lateralization might be the result of brain dysfunction; the poor learning is associated with the dysfunction and not with crossed dominance.

A notable authority who shares this view is Lord Russell Brain[108] (one of the world's leading neurologists), who states: "It is probable that in such cases the failure to establish a dominant hemisphere is the result, and not the cause, of congenital abnormalities of brain function, which also express themselves in disabilities of speech, reading and writing." O. L.

Zangwill,[109] another authority, states that the great majority of poorly lateralized children do not have reading disabilities. He theorizes that a certain proportion of children with ill-defined laterality have, in addition, a slowness in maturation.

It is not the loss of laterality that produces the disorder of language, but if there is a delay in the acquisition of language, most often it is accompanied by other signs of cerebral immaturity, including delayed or incomplete establishment of laterality. The anomaly of handedness is a corollary and not a cause of dyslexia. There is little purpose in using one hand or patching one eye in an effort to establish dominance of one hemisphere.

Of the children who have come to us with reading problems, 65%* have some disturbance in laterality on evaluation of foot, hand, and eye dominance. They might be right-handed and left-eyed, or might have other combinations. Foot and ear seem to be the least significant of the dominance tests. Hand and eye are more significant, with the eye the most significant. Hand preference can be changed by environmental influences more frequently than eye preference, since it is established earlier and more easily recognized as being unusual.

Many surveys have failed to support crossed dominance as a consistent link with reading problems.[110] In a study of a class of 77 pupils who were tested in reading in the first grade and again in the third, 49% of the students favored the right hand and right eye; 30% favored the right hand and left eye; and the remaining 21% exhibited other combinations of hand-eye coordination. Tests on these same children in the third grade revealed that students with mixed eye-hand coordination read as well as students with consistent right-sided dominance. Some children with crossed dominance have no reading difficulties, while others with corresponding laterality exhibit the entire chain of reading difficulties.

Whittey and Kopel[111] in 1936 studied the association between mixed hand and eye dominance with reading disability, and Johnstone[112] also found no correlation between anomalies of lateral dominance and reading disability. Smith[113] in 1950, by matching a group of 50 poor readers with a control group

*This is not a statistically significant figure.

of 50 reading achievers, found no difference between them in hand, foot, ear, and eye preference.

Blind people learning Braille use the left hand, which is most frequently the better sensory receptor.[114] Because the right hemisphere of the brain is most often nondominant and is concerned with spatial relationships, blind persons tend to favor the left hand as their most perceptive hand when reading Braille. This is because they feel the spacings and must use their fingers to judge relationships between raised letters. The blind person rapidly reading Braille "sees" with both his right and left hands. He receives sensory impressions from both the right and left sides of his body at the same time. This compares with the eyes, where such bilateral stimulation is recognized as a phenomenon of retinal rivalry. Unequal retinal rivalry may lead to suppression and amblyopia, but these physiologic disturbances do not result in dyslexia. A child can recognize clues in space with one eye or two, and thus far reversals have not proven to be an abnormality of retinal rivalry.

Benton and McCann[115] reported on a study of 250 patients. They determined the controlling eye through a test of retinal rivalry by using dissimilar targets on the major amblyscope and then counted the number of times that each dissimilar object appeared. Thus they felt that they could differentiate between the dominant or sighting eye and the "controlling eye." The Berners[116] in 1939 introduced this confusing concept of the controlling eye by studying the ocular dominance and handedness of 500 slow readers. The sighting eye is a monocular experience, but the controlling eye is determined in a binocular experience.

The effect of dominance and the controlling eye can best be demonstrated by an illustration of the retinal rivalry phenomenon (See Fig. 11).

A differential may be made between the controlling eye and the dominant eye. The dominant eye is usually the sighting or fixing eye, perhaps selected because it is optically better and therefore produces a clearer image on the retina. However, if the image produced by the dominant eye is significantly reduced by pathology, refractive errors, or any other impediment of focusing, then there could be a transfer for visual control, and the opposite eye would become the "controlling eye." There is

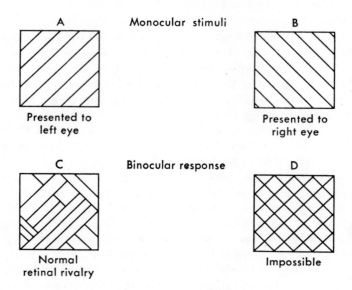

DOMINANCE vs. CONTROLLING EYE

Figure 11. Illustration of retinal rivalry. In A, we expose the left eye to diagonal lines in the right-left direction. In B, we expose the right eye to diagonal lines in the left to right direction. When these stimuli are seen simultaneously, there is no fusion into a cross hatch as in D. What is really seen is an alternating degree of A and B. If ocular control is greater in one eye, more of the pattern from that eye will be similar to C. This is not dependent on dominance.

no immediate shift of the sighting eye, because this is a corticovisuomotor relationship that has been established by years of usage. The controlling eye can be changed by simple changes of refraction.

Reversals and translocation of letters are examples of persistent immaturity not peculiar to dyslexics alone. These errors are notoriously common among all beginners in reading and writing. Usually, however, they are eliminated in the first 2 years of school. Yet the potential for reversals is never eliminated. The adult typist, even a professional typist, continues to make letter reversals when working at high speed or under conditions of stress and fatigue. Proofreading is another example of a persistent reversal tendency. The proofreader misses reversals and translocations in abundance, reading the words as they should be, without seeing errors because his mind has automatically corrected them for him.

The causes of reversals can be summarized as follows: (1) maturational lag, normal in children under the age of five years; (2) lack of auditory and visual feedback; (3) stress (usually emotional) or pressure; (4) pathological sequential disability as in parietal lobe dysfunction; (5) delayed development of handedness and body image.

The dyslexic individual is not unique in making reversals, but he is unique in making so many of them for so long a time. The problems of reversal and translocation are not due to faulty dominance. The confusion can be related to the directional orientation of a symbol, in relationship to the kinesthetic feel of "making" that symbol. For instance, if one closes his eyes and writes the word YOU on a piece of paper held against one's forehead, one can take the card down and see that, almost certainly it has been written UOY. We are so accustomed to writing on a surface facing the eyes that, when we write on a surface that faces away from the eyes, we automatically do this, as if the surface were transparent and the eyes were seeing the message. So, there is some confusion between visual and bodily images which seems to underline some of the difficulties of directional orientation, so characteristic of dyslexics.

The following example will further emphasize and demonstrate that right and left orientation is not only a matter of dominance, but also a matter of normal relationship of visual imagery to kinesthetic imagery: Hold your palms facing you, with the forearms crossed. Keep the wrists crossed and turn the hands so that the palms face each other and lace your fingers into the corresponding interdigital spaces of the other hand. Then, with your eyes closed, have someone touch one finger. You will undoubtedly have some difficulty in recognizing which finger is being touched. In fact, if someone were to touch your index finger, you would first have to start the impulse higher up in the arm and feel the impulse come down the arm and into the finger before you would know exactly which finger you were dealing with.

The more carefully one investigates handedness the more it appears to be a continuous variable. Few adults—and even fewer children—prove to be absolutely right-handed or left-handed. It is true that if a person is right-handed, or claims that he is right-handed, then he will be superior on this right side as compared to the left. But one cannot make the corresponding prediction if an individual states that he is left-handed. A large number of self-classified left-handed individuals show equal or greater preference for the use of the right hand in various activities, as well as equal or greater skill in the right hand.

Ocular dominance cannot be explained by eye anatomy, just as hand dominance cannot be explained by brain anatomy. There is no anatomical arrangement in the eyes themselves, or in their brain connection, that could account for the dominance of, say, the right eye. There is no straightforward anatomical relationship between eye dominance and brain dominance. Shifting the controlling eye can be expected to have little effect upon hand and brain dominance.

Orton,[117] in discussing laterality and reading problems, emphasized the importance of establishing a dominant hemisphere. He claimed that engrams were formed in the associative tracts of both brain hemispheres, but that those in the nondominant hemisphere were not usually employed. If a clear-cut dominance was not established between the two hemispheres, then the engrams of the nondominant side would be mirrorwise. Thus, attempts to change handedness perhaps might result in poor orientation and backwardness in reading.

It has been pointed out time and again that many backward readers are left-handed or poorly lateralized insofar as hand, foot, and eye are concerned. There is a correlation here, but it has yet to be proven what the significance of this correlation is. There was an interesting study by Naidoo, who selected three groups of children, 20 strongly right-handed, 20 strongly left-handed, and 20 with mixed or ambiguous handedness. Tests performed by these children indicated that the mixed group was quite inferior to the two strongly handed groups in the level of verbal intelligence. This mixed group also showed a history of slow speech development and a higher percentage of complications at birth. Perhaps the significance of this correlation might be that there are associated disabilities in poorly lateralized backward readers, which might suggest delayed or incomplete maturation of cerebral functions.

Cerebral maturity and dominance are directly proportional. Children who establish right-handed tendencies early also present the earliest and best-developed signs of general psychomotor maturity. Conversely, cerebral immaturity and poorly differentiated laterality could be directly correlated. The less clearly dominance is established in a given child, the greater are the signs of his general immaturity and the more apt he is to have learning disabilities. The fact that dyslexia seems to have a genetic tendency can be explained by the fact that left-handedness, too, has a genetic tendency. But left-handedness as such cannot be regarded as a simple inversion of right-handedness because there are different types of left-handedness, a genetic and a pathologic form of left-handedness. Finally, in children with poor right-left orientation, it need not only be a matter of cerebral dominance but of a relationship of visual imagery to kinesthetic imagery, sometimes known as body image.

It is agreed that dyslexia is not more frequently present among those children who are poorly lateralized. A lack of definite lateral specialization may imply an atypical cerebral dominance, but atypical cerebral dominance is not characteristic of a large percentage of dyslexics. Dyslexia itself may result from early brain damage or constitutional defects in maturation or retardation secondary to stress, or it may be due to a combination of these and other factors. It should be clear that the solution to problems associated with dyslexia cannot be found simply by changing eye dominance or by laterality training in isolation.[118] Rather, because of the complexity of the problem, an interdisciplinary approach that utilizes the best talent of the various medical disciplines, psychology, and education is essential.

In summary, the notion of cerebral dominance owes its origin to the discovery that a loss of speech almost always results from lesions of the left hemisphere. Inevitably, this suggested a possible link with handedness, and the idea soon gained currency that right-handedness and lateralization of speech were due to an inborn functional preeminence of the left brain hemisphere. In left-handers, it was assumed that the position was exactly reversed. The dominant hemisphere was accepted, with few exceptions, as being contralateral to the preferred hand. This hemisphere was supposed to take the lead in manual skill and dexterity and in the control of articulate speech.

Sufficient evidence has been accumulated to indicate that cerebral dominance and poorly defined laterality are not related to learning disorders. Right-hand preference is usually associated with left cerebral dominance. But left-hand preference does not consistently signify right cerebral hemisphere dominance. Furthermore, dyslexia can occur as a result of a dysfunction in either the major or minor hemisphere.

When dominance of the eye, hand, and foot are inconsistent, and when there might be existing learning difficulties, the presence of the peripheral lack of consistent dominance does not indicate the cause of a learning difficulty, but merely a corollary associated with a central dysfunction or with the etiological factors.

Genetics and Reading Disabilities

The inheritance of man is determined by the information carried in the chromosomes. Forty-six chromosomes are estimated to contain 20,000 to 40,000 different gene pairs, which are subject to variation as a result of mutations of gene structure. Abnormalities in recombination, translocation, and random destribution can further increase the amount of possible variations. Few diseases are either all genetic or entirely environmental in their pathogenesis. Both factors are important and are coordinated. Genetic information can be conveyed by a single chemical reaction which may be under the control of a specific genetic locus. Cell function is under genetic control to a great extent, and mutation of a single gene can result in a structural alteration of the cell, and, if in homozygous dose, the ability of the cell to carry out a single primary chemical reaction can be abolished.

The gene consists of protein material containing an acid—deoxyribonucleic (DNA)—that forms a template on which other nucleic acid molecules of precise structure are synthesized. There are two kinds of nucleic acid: deoxyribonucleic acid (DNA) and ribonucleic acid (RNA). They are chemically similar but functionally different.

Chromosome aberrations responsible for congenital anom-

139

alies were unrecognized in man until recently. These aberrations were not understood until the invention of light microscopy, which permitted the human eye to visualize what had been foreseen 35 years earlier by clinical observation. By cultivation in tissue culture where a sufficient number of cells are stopped in mitosis by addition of colchicine, a sufficient number of metaphases can be observed on a microscopic slide. Five percent of all conceptions carry some form of gross chromosome error.

In man, the primordial germ cell contains 2 sets each of 23 chromosomes, each set inherited from one of the two parents. Except for the XY sex pair in males, each member of a set has its homologue in the other set. At the first division, homologues "recognize" each other and form pairs which exchange genetic material. At fertilization, two cells, each with one set of single chromosomes, fuse to form a zygote, in which the diploid number of chromosomes of the species is restored.

A pictorial display in which an attempt is made to pair homologous chromosomes and to arrange them according to size is called a karyotype. Chromosomes are studied most commonly at the metaphase stage because they are more easily distinguished at that time.

Every chromosome in a normal set can be assigned to one of seven groups labeled A–G, in order of decreasing size. Chromosomal aberrations may be manifested by changes in the structure or number of chromosomes, or both. Diagnosable variations in size, shape, or position, affect multiple systems. Consequently, on reviewing the karyotype, one would not expect to see any abnormality that would be specific for a reading disability alone. Translocation, and others of the numerous possibilities, would lead to greater malformations than would be found in a child with only an auditory or visual memory defect. Therefore, evidence for the genetic inheritance of dyslexia must be obtained from other examinations involving parents, siblings, frequencies, etc., of the individual case history.

Reading disability has been the object of study by investigators from various disciplines, of whom the first were ophthalmologists. Later, neurologists, pediatricians, and educators came into this research field and, during the past 15 years, the experimental psychologist. Recently, much progress has been made in the description, diagnosis, and treatment of the disability. Even though heredity has been cited as a cause for some cases of reading disability, there has been little participation in this research area by the geneticist. Perhaps the two principle reasons for this have been (1) the difficulty in finding adequate tangible evidence that is suitable for genetic analysis, and (2) the problem of reaching agreement on some definitions of reading disability.

Since the control of human behavior is a genetic function, and reading is a behavioral function, then we must look at the evidence for reading disability being a genetic problem. The evidence established thus far involves the following areas: (1) pedigree or family history, (2) the presence of learning disabilities in monozygotic and dizygotic twins, (3) the likelihood that a genetically determined reading disability will persist through a lifetime, (4) the determination of biochemical and chromosomal abberations, and (5) the presence of characteristic abnormal visually evoked responses in family pedigrees.

Critchley[119] believes that it is rare to find a child with dyslexia who does not have a family with one or more similarly afflicted members. Bryant and Patterson[120] assert that, in many cases, probably more than half of their probing interviews would reveal that other family members have also shown a reading disability. Also, although not necessarily a convincing argument for the genetic basis of reading disability, Hallgren[121] has employed genetic statistical techniques in his research, with some convincing results. While an important genetic component of the problem certainly seems to be established, the evidence is not yet conclusive that genetic defect is basic to all reading disability.

Opposed to the idea of the genetic origin of dyslexia is the fact that no chemical or other objective proof that dyslexia is genetically determined has yet been put forward, nor would one expect a biochemical change in a dominant disorder. At a recent conference at the California Institute of Technology on the "Biological Basis of Human Behavior," Childs[122] discussed the genetics of reading disability and indicated that chromosomal abnormalities were not present in these cases.

One of the intriguing problems here is the fact that many of the handicaps which result in defects in a person's ability to process visual or auditory information, or to coordinate and integrate both of these processes, are found in *most* young children who are just beginning to read. In a child with a reading disability, however, these defects persist sometimes for months, sometimes for years, and sometimes for a lifetime. Thus the question arises as to whether or not it is fair to label as "genetic" a handicap present in most children, but one that most can learn to compensate for.

The difficulty in dealing with this question may be seen in the work of Silver and Hagin.[123] They examined 24 persons whom they had observed 10 years earlier as cases of reading disability, and used the same battery of tests on these 24 people. In addition to reading, their methods tested visual-motor, auditory, and tactile functions. The results showed that of the 24 subjects 15 had now become good readers while 9 had not. But, more significantly, they found that the majority still showed the same deficiencies in the nonreading tests that they had shown 10 years earlier. This result suggests that "perceptual training" would have been of no effect, and that there are reasons for thinking that reading disability is sometimes genetically determined.

Bryant and Patterson[124] have pointed out that the hormonal imbalance, suggested by the feminine appearance of boys with reading disability, may or may not be genetically determined. They also indicate that in learning disability two contributors to neurological malfunctioning may be merely mechanisms of genetic determinants. Maturational lag or the slower development of certain cerebral areas (as a genetically influenced development) may be present in many cases of children with reading disability who are immature in size and appearance, and who perform like much younger children.

In looking at a genetic phenotype to submit to analysis, one must consider the various factors involved in reading. Performance, oral and silent reading, spelling, word meaning, perception and spatial patterns, memory of unrelated items, perceptual speed, and other cognitive functions should also be tested. The development of reading skills is dependent in part on the cultural and emotional climate of the immediate family. Thus, if uncles, aunts, and cousins show evidences of reading disability in the same frequency as that found in the index family, the likelihood or origin of the reading problem in cultural or emotional factors is reduced.

The frequency of reading disability is reported as varying from 20% in some school systems to 1 or 2% in others. These numbers differ according to the definitions of reading disability that are applied, and according to whether or not children are included who have not had adequate educational exposure. It would be of considerable interest to study a group incidence involving two or more populations. For example, in Japan, the frequency of reading disability is less than 1%, while the frequency in the United States is 20%. It would be interesting to see what the exposure to reading disability is in a group of Japanese-American children born in this country. It might tell us whether or not the Japanese script is an advantage in learning as opposed to the English sight technique that is practiced in some schools.

Boder[125] described three groups of children: One was defective in phonetic skills, another was deficient in visual perception, and a third group, particularly resistant to treatment, showed deficiencies that were characteristic of both of the first two groups. The source of the defects in all three of these groups could be familial, and Boder suggests that the siblings show the same deficiencies. Three patterns of deficiency were found by Ingram. One group of children had visual-spatial problems, a second group had difficulty in integrating visual and auditory stimuli, while a third group had trouble comprehending words or sentences and in recalling appropriate words to express ideas. Because of the diversity of the symptomatology of all of these cases, it is just not likely that the genes would be the same for all of them.

Critchley[127] feels that to blame some environmental factor for learning disability is not likely to be correct since the evidence, in many cases, goes back generation to generation. The evidence for a genetic cause for specific reading disability was first noted because of the familial aggregations of cases of specific reading disability; the conclusion was made that therefore there must be a hereditary form of it. The data favoring this hypothesis were of three kinds: (1) family history and pedigree analysis, (2) concordance of single-ovum twins, and (3) other characteristic.

One of the difficulties in pedigree analysis is that there may be one sibling who may have a similar disability, and it may appear that the parents or relatives have had a similar disability. But, very frankly, no one has taken the trouble to examine the parents, relatives, and siblings of the child with the reading disability. The fact that a family group has many instances of learning disability does not prove a genetic origin. It may be accounted for by the common cultural environment experienced by members of the family.

Actually, there has been only one major genetic study, and that one was done by Hallgren,[128] who examined 116 retarded readers and discovered 160 secondary cases in their families. Hallgren did extensive physical examinations and gave informal reading and spelling tests to the parents and to a few other adult relatives. He concluded that primary dyslexia is a dominant characteristic. Hallgren found no consistent relationship between reading disabilities and handedness. In the families, although there were slightly more males affected then females, the difference in instance by sex was much smaller than that found among the usual reported case histories.

Hermann[129] has studied 45 sets of twins, of whom at least one twin had a reading disability. Twelve pairs of these twins were one-egg (monozygotic) or identical twins, and in all twelve pairs both twins showed identical disability. Thirty-three sets of these twins were two-egg (dizygotic) or nonidentical. Nineteen of these sets of two-egg twins were of the same sex, but in only four sets did both twins have reading disability. Fourteen sets were opposite-sex twins and in only seven sets did both twins have reading disability. Thus, in the one-egg twins there was a 100% concordance of disability, while in the two-egg twins there was only 33% concordance. These findings would *indicate* that dyslexia is genetically determined and not dependent on environmental influences. It is commonly observed that any genetically determined characteristic persists for life, while variations due to developmental change disappear in time and those due to injury may be overcome by healing processes. If there is a genetic cause of some cases of reading disability, then one must realize that, just as inborn errors of metabolism are never outgrown, the appropriate treatment is one that rearranges the environment so as to allow the affected person to tolerate his disability. This relates directly to the work of Margaret Rawson,[130] who interviewed and followed patients who had dyslexia for 20 years. She found that, although the educational attainments of these people were no less than those of normal readers, many of them continued to find reading and spelling an embarrassing task.

In summary, there are some reasons for believing that reading disability can be genetically determined. Familial groupings of cases do exist. The observation of reading difficulties in twins, especially identical twins, is strongly suggestive of a genetic origin. The persistence of the reading deficiency characteristic into adult life in some persons is also compatible with the genetic hypothesis.

The multiplicity of causes of the reading-disability characteristic and the diagnostic imprecision involved pose some problems. Before a genetic etiology can be proven, there must be much better evidence of heredity and the possibility of genetic heterogeneity. A child may have different genes which provoke different symptoms, such as finger agnosia, memory difficulty, or a visual-perceptual difficulty. Yet, each one of these difficulties can produce a learning disability.

The appropriate use of genetic analysis, together with the broadening of the set of phenotype characteristics to be tested should include neurophysiological and biochemical attributes, and should tell us whether or not reading disabilities are genetically determined, how many hereditary types there are, and perhaps the frequency of the genes that cause them. Of course, this mode of attack upon the problem of reading disability may be of questionable importance or, even, merely academic. Since we are not going to have selective breeding of human beings, we are still going to have to try to deal with the child who is unable to achieve, who becomes frustrated, and is resentful and disturbed.

Children with dyslexia can succeed, as evidenced by the history of numerous individuals such as Winston Churchill, Harvey Cushing, Thomas Edison, Albert Einstein, Paul Ehrlich, George Patton, Auguste Rodin, and Woodrow Wilson. All of these individuals and others have been classified as dyslexics, yet they have enjoyed successful lives and careers.

The Chemistry of Learning and Drug Therapy

It is now clear that learning should no longer be thought of in terms of some simple relationship between stimulus and response or stimulus-response reinforcement. Recent studies on the chemistry of the brain have shown that learning and thinking are processes vastly more complex than traditional learning theory had suggested. Learning seems to involve a number of highly sophisticated and complicated processes, including acquisition of information, processing of information, establishment of memory, maintenance of memory, and retrieval of information. Memory itself is divided into its long-term and short-term aspects, both involving enormously complex processes in the brain. Short-term memory appears to be electrical-neurological in nature, but long-term memory clearly involves biochemical processes.

Since learning and memory seem to be composed of specific and discrete sets of processes or functions, this new view suggests to some, for example, the idea that mental retardation is not a single, all-encompassing phenomenon. Rather, it is possible to think of it in terms of defects which exist in specific functions, such as acquisition of information, memory formation, or memory retention. The recent discoveries about the chemistry of the brain indicate that, if we are to understand how learning really takes place, we will have to comprehend the inordinately complicated process of interaction between heredity, development, and environment that constantly goes on in the brain.

It seems clear that the environment (through experience) produces chemical changes in the brain. But one cannot understand how the brain responds to an environmental input without some understanding of its particular genetic makeup. Some human behaviors, for instance, are apparently innate, precoded or preprogrammed into the brain. Learned behavior, at this point in our knowledge, does not seem to differ greatly from innate behavior, and this suggests that the chemical processes governing both innate and learned behavior must be the same.

One known fact is that experience, notably the experience of learning, demonstrably and literally changes the chemistry of the brain. Experiments involving both trained and untrained rats have found both chemical and anatomical changes in the brains of the trained rats, including a heavier brain cortex, more glial cells, more enzyme activity, and a superior blood supply to the brain. Other experimental work along these lines has found that the act of learning sets a specific biochemical process into motion, which alters the protein-RNA* structure of the brain in a specific way. In trained rats, new fractions of RNA appear in the nerve cells of the brain. Thus, the crucial biochemical process in learning appears to involve a change in the way the brain synthesizes protein and RNA.

This relationship can work both ways. By changing the biochemical functioning of the brain, one seems to be able to change an animal's ability to learn or remember. Experiments with trained goldfish, conducted by Agranoff,[131] at the University of Michigan, utilized injections of a chemical which suppresses protein synthesis. If injected into the brain within an hour after learning, the learning is destroyed; if the injection is delayed more than an hour, memory is not affected and the learned action can still be performed. Agranoff's work suggests that the *formation* of long-term memory requires protein synthesis in the brain, while the *maintenance* of long-term memory

*Ribonucleoprotein: a giant molecule formed from a particular kind of nucleic acid and protein.

does not. It also suggests that long-term memory is formed by protein synthesis in the brain within a specific period of time—in this case, 1 hour.

A number of researchers have posed this question: If the formation of memory is dependent upon RNA-mediated protein synthesis, could memory (and learning) be enhanced by chemically stimulating such synthesis? McGaugh at the University of California has found that learning and long-term memory appear to be greatly facilitated by a drug injection in rats taught to run a maze. He has also found that other drugs either enhance or suppress short-term memory, without affecting long-term memory. A drug manufactured by a national pharmaceutical laboratory is now being clinically tested in human beings to determine its value as a performance booster. Some preliminary results indicate that it may enhance memory in pre-senile adults, but other reports were negative. Much more experimental work will have to be done before any conclusion can be reached, but it is evident now that many research chemists believe that it may soon be possible to increase a human being's capacity for learning through drugs.

The implications of all this for education will remain tentative because the present knowledge of the brain and of its chemistry is still incomplete. Nevertheless, research in this field is proceeding rapidly and many who are involved in it expect a breakthrough within the next 10 years. When a coherent picture of brain mechanisms does emerge, it will have enormous implications for education and for the learning process. Indeed, some feel that eventually there may be a whole arsenal of drugs, each affecting a different part of the learning process. It may be awesome to contemplate the educational and social consquences of this, depending upon the possibilities that emerge. Some anticipate that drugs can be found which will raise IQ levels by 10 points all across the spectrum. Others expect only to increase the capacity of those at the bottom end of the IQ scale. Some think now that the *rate* at which people learn can be greatly quickened by drugs, while others foresee the human *capacity* to learn as being increased as well.

For those with learning disabilities, the implications for the use of "learning drugs" are equally tentative. In addition to what is still unknown about learning and the biochemical processes of the brain, too little is still known about the causes of learning disability. These are certainly all tied together to some extent, and research findings in one area may help to unravel the mysteries in the other areas. For the time being, at least, drug utilization in cases of learning disability will probably be limited to individual cases and to specific types of problems.

As incredible as it seems, the early grades of the public schools in some areas are already encountering cases of drug usage in children as young as eight or nine years. In such cases, their learning problems are sometimes a cause of drug usage and sometimes a result of it. Because of this contemporary development, those with a concern for learning and the educational process should give some serious attention to its implications.

Among the causes of drug usage that have been found to relate to learning problems are (1) academic pressures, (2) intolerable slum and ghetto living conditions, and (3) a reinforcement for the defiance of authority (at school or at home, or both). In the student world, there is a widespread belief that the use of amphetamines (which reduce the sleep span) will increase the study span and the brain's capacity for sorting and storing information. Of course, this is a myth; actually, while they do stimulate activity in normal, well-rested persons, the amphetamines do so in an uncoordinated way and really reduce rather than increase memory storage. Slum and ghetto youth use a variety of drugs to relieve the pains of terrible home and living conditions, aiming for a feeling of euphoria. Drug abuse is a means of withdrawing from school problems as well. The student who is failing, who has become convinced that he is stupid and lazy, may also turn to illicit drugs. For some, it may be withdrawal from problems; for others, it may be a means of challenging and defying parents, the teacher, or the society in which he is a failure; and for some it may be the lure of a promised "mind expansion" that will solve his learning difficulties.

Doubtless there are many other reasons why children resort to drugs. Whether they do so because of academic failure or whether academic failure results from their drug abuse, these children create classroom problems of great magnitude and they damage their own bodies and the delicate chemical processes of the brain. For example, the morphine-type drugs produce a variety of pathological results, even death. The use of nonsterile needles and contaminated doses of such drugs can result in hepatitis, tetanus, uremia, brain damage, and heart damage. Marijuana in very large doses can induce changes in brain function as great as those produced by heroin and LSD. If the experimentation with drugs by children in the lower grades continues to grow, we may be confronted with large numbers of cases of learning disability that have been induced by drug usage.

In children, profound behavioral changes result from a psychological dependence on drugs. The use of "hard drugs" (opium, heroin, morphine, cocaine, and certain barbiturates that are depressants) show effects that range from severe depression and irrational irritation to overexcitement, rage, and uncontrolled violence in the absence of the drug. Some drugs, on the other hand, produce completely apathetic children. Where a physiological dependence has been established, the absence of the drug leads to a wide range of familiar "withdrawal" symptoms, such as perspiration, dilated pupils with blurred vision, and nausea. Because these drugs are illegal, various aspects of antisocial behavior are associated with the attitudes and actions of the users. Removed from the normal structure of social relations, the drug user usually joins the drug subculture, which has its own rules of conduct.

Because many important biochemical, neurophysiological, and general physiological factors are involved in the learning process, it should be evident that drugs and chemical compounds represent a significant and potentially critical intervention in that process. Where drug use is generally illicit and self-administered, the prognosis is not good for learning or the classroom situation. However, for a number of problems associated with learning and with learning diability, therapeutic drug intervention can often be beneficial. This involves the use of carefully selected drugs, prescribed and administered by the appropriate medical practitioner. To deal with a child's current learning difficulty, it may be necessary to pursue a specific program of drug administration in order to alter beneficially his learning pattern. Of course, this is usually a temporary expedient; in the long run, a reliance upon behavioral manipulation by drugs is ordinarily unsound.

No drug should be used without some firm indication that its use may be helpful. Not all poor readers show improvement with drug therapy, but some do. Further, it is hoped that when a drug is used, the doses will become progressively smaller until there can be a discontinuance of it. This occurs when the child is able to rely upon himself rather than upon drugs for successful attention and controlled hyperactivity in class.

In discussing therapeutic intervention of drugs in the learning problems of children, it should be stressed that drugs ought not be used empirically. Three groups of children should be identified. First, there are the children who have minimal neurological signs (brain damage) and positive EEG findings. A child in this category is best controlled by the use of drugs, such as Dilantin. The next group of children consists of the emotionally disturbed. A tranquilizer would be the best treatment for a child in this group, and the recommended tranquilizer would be Thorazine. The third group of children who would be responsive to drug therapy is composed of those who are hyperactive and for whom Ritalin would be generally benefical.

In discussing hyperactivity in children, one must be careful to differentiate between hyperactivity and the results of plain parental permissiveness. There are a number of children who are hyperactive and restless. They are demanding, have temper tantrums, and show short attention spans for the things they do not like. The neurological examination of such a child can show him to be normal, but the parents will make no effort to discipline him. As they go along with his every demand and whim, he, in turn, remains in a preschool stage, retaining an impulsiveness pattern that is normally characteristic only for preschool children. After such a child gets into the upper grades in school, he has more and more difficulty. When the teacher begins to set limits on his behavior, the child becomes a disciplinary problem. This type of immature impulsiveness does not usually disappear. As a result, there are many children who do not learn well and do not do satisfactory work in school because they have never been required to discipline themselves in any way.

The use of drugs to control such undisciplined children is not recommended because they offer no possibility of providing what is most needed for a permanent remedy. Where only discipline and self-discipline can permanently change the behavior of such children, the use of drugs as a substitute only delays the application of the cure. In fact, one should never try to prescribe drug therapy for a child whose symptoms might stem from a correctible social, familial, biological, or interpersonal disturbance. Resorting to the use of drugs without strenuous efforts to remove these causative factors should be avoided.

In a minority of children with learning disorders, certain stimulant drugs do improve a number of their cognitive and behavioral functions, especially their attention. Stimulant drugs enhance the state of alertness of the child, which in turn affects the state of arousal of the brain's cortex and its inhibitory functions. There is some weak evidence that stimulants may improve short-term memory, and in some children they may control hyperactive aggressive behavior. Stimulants such as the amphetamines or methylphenidate should be tried wherever there is a combination of a behavioral and a learning problem which does not yield to a simpler method. After the child has reached the age of 12, however, stimulant drugs should not be used.

The group of drugs known as phenothiazines may produce what is perceived by adults as improvement. However, there is increasing and compelling evidence that phenothiazines and similar tranquilizers actually depress the learning function. The child may *appear* to improve because he is quieter, but there is also the possibility that there may be a depression of intellect. These tranquilizers are recommended for use only when the child is extremely disruptive and when he has not responded to the stimulant medications. Barbiturates are not recommended at all, because they seem actually to contribute to a deterioration of behavior.

The only way to find out whether a drug work successfully in learning and behavioral problems is to try it. This presupposes a thorough medical examination of the child, including complete physiological and neurological findings. In this way, the child who is simply undisciplined and the child who is on a self-administered drug can be isolated. The main advantage is that the medical examiner can better determine the type of drug therapy that promises the most beneficial results.

Drug therapy should not be sought lightly by parents. Drugs should be prescribed only where they will help the patient, not to appease his parents. The most common side effects of drug therapy are loss of appetite, insomnia, irritability, sadness, nausea, headaches, cramps, and jitters. Once undertaken, drug therapy should follow a very good principle: If the dosage has been pushed to the point where side effects occur and there is still doubt as to whether or not the drug is effective, then it is not effective and it should be discontinued.

Laymen and professional people alike will do well, in their involvement in the learning problems of children, to be more aware of the potential dangers in administering drugs to children. The indiscriminate and unsupervised administration of tranquilizers in the home or classroom to children who manifest behavioral and/or learning problems is a form of Russian roulette. Where these problems exist, drug therapy should be administered by a physician or someone acting upon his orders, directed toward a specific strategy of correction of the disorder, and constantly supervised. It is the medical doctor who is best able to determine what drug to employ, how long to employ it, and in what dosage to use it. He is best able to judge its effectiveness. Any amateur practice of drug therapy runs the risk of inflicting damage that is both psysiologically and neurologically irreparable in the child.

Education Prevention and Remediation

During the last decade there has been a tremendous increase in interest at the national, state, and local level, in the development of programs for disabled readers. Medical, paramedical, and educational specialists are making every effort to develop techniques to differentiate between achieving and non-achieving readers. However, as diagnostic and remediation techniques become more sophisticated, the number of identified disabled readers is not decreasing. In fact, the truth of the matter is that many previously unidentified disabilities are being uncovered and longer waiting lists for available resources are resulting. Ideally, these pupils would be identified and helped in the regular classroom by proper grouping. However, from experience we know this is not always possible or practical. Very often it is necessary that special reading programs be available at the elementary and secondary level to supplement the developmental program. Emphasis should be placed upon early identification and placement in the proper program before an individual's problem has become too complex.

A total school reading program must involve at least three kinds of reading: developmental, corrective, and remedial. The developmental phase involves systematic instruction at all school levels and in all content areas for those who are developing language abilities commensurate with their general capacity levels. This developmental phase is the responsibility of every teacher, affects all the pupils, is provided for in the regular curriculum, and is a continuous on-going process.

The corrective phase of reading must deal with those pupils who are able to comprehend the assigned material only after undue and laborious effort. Many difficulties involved are those common to all pupils in reading, but are greatly accentuated. Most of the corrective instruction is the responsibility of all teachers in their daily class activities. In some school systems, a special reading teacher provides systematic instruction in small-group situations.

The remedial phase of reading usually involves a small clinical group showing severe symptoms of reading retardation. These children may differ from those in the corrective area by the degree and type of their deficiency; and the cases are frequently complicated by severe personality problems, defects in special mental capacities, and physical handicaps. These pupils demand individual attention, special methods, and a highly trained, clinically oriented teacher. It is often in this last group that reading difficulty may result in a real damage to pupil personality. A child who cannot read, or who cannot read as well as his group, is marked before all as a failure—a failure he is reminded of many times a day, every day. Even a considerate teacher cannot in most cases restore his confidence in himself since his classmates and parents often magnify his deficiency.

Unfortunately there are administrative problems involved in executing recommendations for the treatment of severe reading disorders within most on-going educational systems.

These difficulties may be organized under four major headings:

(1) Defining the problem.
(2) Administrative and educational inertia.
(3) Organization of the program.
(4) Evaluation and research.

Defining the Problem

One of the basic problems is that we cannot agree on what we are talking about. First, there is no agreement on the definition or name for the disorder. Some educators refer to the problem category as *remedial, strephosymbolia, associative learning disability, specific reading or language disability, congenital word blindness, primary reading retardation, or developmental dyslexia.* To avoid semantic confusion we must agree on the name. One school district may refer to all retarded readers as *remedial;* another agency, in the same community, may use the term *remedial* for the small group of children with specific learning difficulties.

Our next problem is defining the term. Most of the current definitions are expressed in terms of specific etiology or measurable performance. Definitions cover heredity, organic, congenital, psychogenic, social, and educational causes, and may include all pupils who are more than two years retarded in reading according to grade level, or only the children with "associative learning problems." No one has been able to clearly validate the two-year cutoff, let alone to agree on how to measure grade-level achievement. Standardized tests of ability and achievement are more suspect every day. The latest definition that defines the dyslexic as one who cannot learn to read by conventional techniques or conventional school organization is quite different from the definition that states that the disorder is totally organic in nature. In fact, another semantic "hang-up" has developed since educators have never been able to agree on a definition for the word *conventional.* Because of this lack of agreement, we cannot even guess at the number of pupils involved. Experts quote figures from half of 1% to 20% of the total school population.

In summary, the first barrier simply revolves around lack of communication. We must agree, no matter how arbitrary the decision, on a name and a practical functional definition for this disability. *This must be done before we can accurately determine the frequency and the etiology.* The solution to all other barriers is based on first solving this problem.

Administrative and Educational Inertia

Administrators often do not understand what the problem is—namely, that there are such a large number of children who have not been successful learners with the traditional methods. Too often, only lip service has been given to the "individual" child, "individualization" of programs, etc., but in reality children are lined up, educationally spray-gunned, and, then, if that does not take, the pupil is a "problem."

Some of the educational practices that are barriers towards implementing a dyslexia program are as follows:

1. The traditional three reading groups.

2. Administrative decisions that notify teachers in September what page in the book they must reach by February.

3. Principals' comments that we cannot expect teachers to know what all the learning problems are along with "everything else we expect them to do."

4. Educational decisions to categorize pupils as problems if they do not learn by the standard methods of approach that are successful with most children.

Of course, the fact that any effective dyslexia program will be very expensive is also a deterrent. Providing sufficient space, extra personnel, teacher training, and special materials costs money. An effective program may take years to prove successful. If administrators are not completely sold on the program, they may fear that they are doing something just too unorthodox and expensive. Pressure from board members and the public can build rapidly and the tendency to look for a speedy magic panacea can become overwhelming.

The real problem may be that the decision-making personnel are often too far removed from the classroom to observe the failures and to search for newer ideas about the causes. The great number of committees through which ideas have to be forced in order to finally be accepted, and the danger of dilution and modification after the idea has been exposed to these committees, is a serious factor in large school districts. It is difficult for anyone removed from day-to-day contact with children to be highly motivated about the seemingly small ideas and creative approaches that actually help children. People removed from interaction with pupils should be concerned with the administration of the program after the ideas have been proven to be effective. It is unfair to expect people who are not in constant contact with children to be very creative in things that affect youngsters directly.

In summary, a major problem is the lack of knowledge and understandings on the part of administrators. Innovation is difficult for many experienced educators, and inertia will inhibit experimentation and the development of new programs. Unfortunately, I do not believe that any effective program can be developed without administrative approval and leadership.

Organization of the Program

If the school system has defined the population they want to consider in their dyslexia program, and if the educators can agree on the basic philosophy for implementation, the next barrier is the actual organization and administration of the remediation program.

1. Structure of the Remediation Program

A decision must be made on what type of organizational program should be provided for these pupils, such as assistance in the regular classroom, small-group and one-to-one tutoring program, or a full-time clinic. Frequently, different departments (i.e. general instruction versus special education) develop empire-building conflicts that can retard the growth and development of the program. The prevalent attitude among many semi-informed and concerned educators (but this attitude is fortunately changing) is that the dyslexic child is so special that he must receive special placement, thereby implying the necessity of removal from even a modified program of studies. Unfortunately, with this philosophy in mind, a child labeled "dyslexic" may sit and vegetate in a regular classroom while waiting for admission to a special program. The classroom teacher becomes so terrified by the diagnosis that she avoids contact with the disabled reader. If the educators become too fearful and concerned, the hopelessness which they feel in trying to help might result in their "standing still" until they can afford to establish a clinic. Although a reduced class size, individual instruction, or interdisciplinary clinic would undoubtedly be ideal, the situation can be greatly helped within the regular classroom structure with appropriate techniques. Of course, whenever possible, there is a need for one-to-one and small-group teaching for the most severe cases and for those pupils who have reached upper grade placement and have not received proper treatment.

A basic premise of remedial teaching is that each child

needs to work on his own developmental level. This level may be different for each area of learning. In grouping the children, their levels of education and social development must be taken into account. However, if the children do get grouped, the only factors taken into consideration will probably be decoding, speed, and comprehension. It is difficult to see any real change in the teaching approach. The top group does what the bottom group does—only faster. Where does this leave the child with excellent comprehension but faulty decoding ability? Where does this leave the child with both faulty comprehension and decoding? Unfortunately, it usually leaves him in the *same* reading group, using the *same* techniques as the top group— only moving at a snail's pace.

2. Early Identification

The literature underscores quite clearly the importance of early identification of children with reading disabilities. It was noted in an earlier chapter that within a prescribed 2-year treatment period approximately 80% of the second-grade children were remediated in contrast to a 6% remediation of ninth-grade pupils. More important than the number of cases remediated, however, is the quality of the remediation. Research conducted in the spring of 1969 suggests that children remediated in the secondary schools have difficulty maintaining their skills and achievement levels when returned to the regular classroom program. This same degree of remission does not occur in the elementary grades.

One of the major problems inherent in the identification of reading disabilities is that traditionally educators, physicians, and other professional workers concerned with the problem have relied almost exclusively on capacity and achievement scores determined by standardized tests. Standardized tests of reading achievement do not always indicate the pupil's optimal instructional reading level.

Standardized tests may be used to test individuals or groups. These tests have norms, and the achievement scores can be compared with the scores of people all over the country. Standardized tests measure a multitude of specific skills, abilities, and information that are crucial in reading situations. These tests are developed to serve different purposes; no single test can measure adequately the entire reading facet of language development. One tends to overlook the fact that standardized tests may be expected to measure "frustration levels" in reading, and possibly can range from one to four levels above the point at which instruction can be profitably begun. The reason lies in the fact that a reader does not have to read every word in an exercise in order to mark the example correctly, and that there are many opportunities for guessing. Students should not be pigeon-holed at one reading level on the basis of a single test score.

Informal tests may also be used to gain some insight into the nature and degree of the reading problem. Informal tests are usually designed by teachers and usually have no norms. They are primarily clinical instruments that have been adapted for limited classroom use. Informal reading inventories and word-recognition tests fit into this category.

Careful observation during instruction by the experienced teacher is still the most practical classroom method for evaluating reading problems.

The picture is just as confusing concerning capacity evaluations. Most of the measuring instruments are tests that require reading, yet often they are given to students who cannot read or who have not learned to read effectively. There is considerable variability among the different capacity-measuring instruments.

It is more difficult but very necessary to identify as early as the kindergarten levels potentially dyslexic children and begin teaching them appropriately in the first grade. Most of the present first-grade evaluation programs are not interpreted in a manner that identifies such children. Thus, we have no idea how many children we are talking about until they are in the third grade. By then, the problem has changed from a preventive one to a remedial and emotional one. Sometimes a dyslexic child is intelligent enough to memorize enough vocabulary to avoid being considered a remedial case until the fourth grade. However, the cutoff grade in his school may be the third grade because of the school's concern and concentration on early remediation. If the child is lucky he may be seen twice a week. By then even the most intelligent child may need a minimum of 1 hour a day and probably needs it on an individual basis.

Very often administrators cannot accept this one-to-one relationship and assign their "expensive" reading specialist to large groups of pupils instead of small groups of dyslexics.

While it is generally not too difficult for trained people working with dyslexic children to be able to identify them, it does require many disciplines working together in order to distinguish them from the organic or emotionally disturbed groups. Interdisciplinary teams can be very helpful in this area. Unfortunately, when medical and paramedical personnel work with teachers another problem arises—the problem of interdisciplinary communication. Very often each discipline sees the child in terms of his own specialization. Everyone becomes a piece worker, and the resultant mosaic is sometimes quite different from the original child. Another problem arises in addition to the communication difficulty. For years, educators have considered the responsibility of teaching reading the province of the elementary teacher. Considerable re-education will be necessary for effective interdisciplinary cooperation. Very often a good public relations job is needed to unite the program with regular classroom teachers, administrators, medical and paramedical personnel, and parents. Generally, parental objection is not an obstacle. Parents usually are most anxious to cooperate when properly educated and informed.

3. Space

Unfortunately, there is frequently the lack of necessary space within the school for instituting the small-group or clinical program. Enough rooms for the necessary one-to-one or very-small-group teaching are hard to find—sometimes even one small room is unavailable.

4. Staff

Additional numbers of staff positions would be necessary in each school—both in the number of specialized instructors and/or remediators, and in supportive services. Volunteers and aides can make a valuable contribution if properly trained. In addition, however, teachers must also be taught how effectively to employ the supplementary personnel.

5. Material

The problem of limited or ineffective materials and method guidelines in all other subject areas in addition to reading is considerable. Some adaptation of content curriculum for the dyslexic children is an imperative. If pupils receive adequate therapy in language arts but meet frustration in other subjects, the total remediation program will suffer considerably. This frustration is particularly noticeable and acute in grades 9–12. Usually, the minimum number of Carnegie units required for high-school graduation is 18, of which 12 must be in the field of general education. Dyslexic pupils may not be able to obtain the 12 units if they are not in the regular school program and will be denied the opportunity to be graduated. Some adjustment must be made in these Carnegie requirements.

6. Teacher Education

One of the major barriers to implementing a meaningful dyslexic program is the difficulty in obtaining qualified teachers. Many neophyte teachers coming out of teacher training colleges do not understand the concepts and basic skills necessary for teaching a successful reading program. The problem of inadequately trained teachers is more pressing because it involves a serious difference of opinion among educators of teacher training institutions. The argument as to whether to emphasize subject-matter courses or professional-techniques courses has been going on for some time. The subject-matter proponents appear to be in the ascendency. Local universities offer the most minimal undergraduate training in the myriad approaches to the teaching of reading. In fact, a secondary school teacher of English or language arts can be graduated from most teacher training schools in the country without ever having taken a course in the teaching of reading. The average primary school teacher may be required to take one course in the teaching of reading or language arts.

To complicate matters, a large number of certified employed teachers have never had a college course in teaching reading, and many who have had a course do not appear to really understand the basic language-arts concepts. The situation becomes of greater concern when we face the fact that in most systems we are teaching reading by many different methods and that local schools change these methods from year to year. In addition, the schools often have not agreed upon one systematic sequence of skills. This lack of an organized and accepted sequence of skills for all children and the switching from one pedagogical procedure or material to another causes innumerable problems for our inexperienced and experienced teachers alike.

In the area of dyslexia, the problem is a hundred times worse. Very few colleges even recognize the condition, let alone offer courses in the area at the undergraduate or graduate level. If educators cannot change the requirements or philosophies of the teacher training institutions, then the local school systems must provide an on-going program of in-service education and curriculum development. In other words, schools will not only need to teach children but also to teach teachers.

Most present in-service programs consist of releasing teachers 5 or 6 days during the school year. This approach has not effectively trained teachers to deal with the dyslexic child.

Another type of traditional in-service training where master teachers demonstrate techniques with small groups of pupils and national authorities lecture on the finest pedagogical procedures is also of questionable value. One sees a lot of enthusiasm and interest generated, but very little change or impact in the classroom.

Theoretically, staff can be trained during the summer. However, this is difficult to implement since most local units cannot afford massive in-service programs. In-service teacher education, so desperately needed, can be conducted effectively at the local-school level during the school day. Many administrators reject this concept of released time since it takes considerable planning and organization. Also, if local systems are going to train their own teachers, they must find instructors who understand the uniqueness of the dyslexic child and the unusual way in which he learns the language.

The secondary schools, by proper scheduling, can release a small number of teachers throughout the school day for their in-service program. For example, all seventh-grade science teachers might be free the third period on Tuesdays. When all teachers in one subject area cannot be free at one time, in-service meetings can be conducted with a group of teachers from several subject-matter areas. This latter type of in-service session, with its rich interaction, is often more valuable and meaningful for everyone involved.

Elementary school scheduling is a little more difficult to arrange. However, several schools in at least one county are already using their special teachers, volunteers, and aides in back-to-back scheduling for releasing their classroom teachers several hours a week for in-service and planning time. Time can be arranged at local school levels for effective in-service by the proper scheduling of professional staff.

One elementary school arranged its in-service schedule in the folowing manner. For each school-wide age group, there is a teaching team consisting of teachers and teacher aides. The size of the team is determined by the number and age level of pupils. In each team, one of the teachers has the responsibility for being the team leader. The team as a whole, under the leadership of the team leader, plans the instructional activities for each of the units of instruction. From 8:30 AM to 9:30 AM on Mondays and Thursdays, the teams at the primary level meet to review the instructional activities planned for that week. On Tuesdays and Fridays the teams at the intermediate level meet. From 9:00 AM to 9:30 AM, the pupils whose teachers are meeting assemble in the multipurpose room for morning exercises, general announcements, and some appropriate program. The planning for this half-hour is the responsibility of the principal.

One half-day each week is set aside for discussion by the team on the progress being made by pupils and of particular pupil problems. This half-day is also used to plan instructional activities. During the half-day, pupils are in meetings for various types of activities such as student council, school landscape clubs, interest clubs, and activities growing out of classroom experiences. These activities are planned by the special teachers—e.g., teachers of music and physical education—in a team with the principal as team leader and the librarian as coordinator. The sessions are conducted by interested and competent parents and members of community civic groups, such as historical societies and garden clubs.

The coordination of the entire school's instructional program is the responsibility of the principal through the team leaders. The principal also has the responsibility for assisting the teachers and teacher aides in their professional growth, aided by the consultant service of the central-staff personnel.

It is difficult to arrange this in-service time, but it can be done. All elementary and secondary schools are urged to plan their programs and schedules in such a way that released time will be available to teachers during the school day for in-service and staff planning.

Although the in-service programs will depend upon the needs of the local school, one basic philosophy should be stressed in all subject matter and for all grade levels. School personnel should not dissipate their time, energy, and funds looking for the one best method of teaching reading or arguing about the advantages of teaching phonics vs. the whole-word method. Each teacher must be trained to select material and curriculum that meet the needs and skills of the pupils. For example, if an author, Dr. X, writes a selection for fourth-grade pupils, he assumes that his reader brings to the reading situation a certain number of prerequisites. Among other things, he assumes that the pupil has a certain background of information, a certain vocabulary strength, a certain number of working concepts, and a certain interest. Dr. X, the author, does not know Miss Y, the teacher, nor does he know Miss Y's pupils. He writes this selection based on mythical pupils or students with whom he has come in contact through his teaching experience. Miss Y is the only one who really knows her fourth-grade pupils. She knows the skills and strengths that they bring to the learning situation. She must decide if her pupils have the prerequisites that the author desires. If they do not, then she must have the authority to reject the material or take time to develop sufficient readiness. This readiness pace cannot be predetermined by the teacher's manual, course of study, or an administrator. This is as true for a twelfth-grade science class as for a first-grade language arts program.

7. Pedagogical Procedures

A corps of reading specialists should be available to all school personnel for specific consultations regarding problems that the reading and study skills teachers and other specialists at the local level cannot handle. Further, an interdisciplinary team composed of medical, paramedical, psychological, and educational personnel will identify children with severe reading disabilities who cannot learn to read with conventional techniques or conventional school organizations. These children may be transferred to Specific Learning Problems Centers. Since the literature is so confused concerning the "dyslexic, strephosymbolic, word blind, remedial, SLD" child, it may be of some value to explain this program.

The children in these centers are functioning on an educationally retarded level. All of them have specific learning disabilities such as visual-motor problems, auditory-perception problems, difficulty in dealing with symbols, impaired body image, spatial disorientation, figure-ground disturbance, impaired gross or fine motor skills, or other problems of language and communication. Some of the children have obvious physical problems such as cerebral palsy, epilepsy, hearing and speech defects, lack of visual acuity, and congenital handicaps. Many also have obvious behavioral problems. They are excitable, easily confused or distracted, and require a great deal of personal attention from their teachers. They all give indication of either being neurologically impaired or behaving as if they were neurologically impaired. The children usually have difficulty in more than one of these areas: physiological, learning, and bebehavior. It therefore becomes necessary to determine which is the area of primary involvement that needs to be worked with before further learning can take place. When a specific learning problem can be defined, individualized teaching methods, materials, and techniques are utilized to help these children to circumvent or to overcome their particular learning disabilities. How early the child with the learning problem is referred for help, and whether or not there is an organic basis for the problem, are two of the important factors affecting the amount of progress the child can expect to make.

The pupil-teacher ratio is 7–10 children per teacher. One aide assists the teachers. Experience at this center seems to indicate that the program functions best with a maximum of 50 children. The children stay at this center for 1–3 years. During this time, close contact is maintained with other people who are working with each child. Evaluation conferences involving the faculty, supervisors, pupil personnel worker, public health nurse, and others are held at least once a year to consider the growth, development, future plans, and placement for each child. Conferences are also held during the school year whenever a child is not benefiting from the program because he has needs that this center is not equipped to provide.

The role of this center is to develop and to improve the communication skills of each child. Because of neurological impairment, some of the children come with no usable language, some with severely disorganized language, and some with confused language patterns. Therefore, it is necessary that the staff stabilize, as far as possible, the language and concepts used with each child. For example, before the concept of likenesses and differences is introduced in the visual perception program, the teachers discuss and agree upon the exact vocabularly and the question form that will be used. At the same time the concept is being developed in visual perception, it is also introduced in the auditory-perception program. The music and physical education teachers use the same concepts in their programs.

For those individuals with specific reading disabilities, special methods are necessary. Many are able, however, to develop good reading abilities. To do this they must use, for word learning, techniques which allow them to use tactile and/or kinesthetic clues as well as visual and auditory. VAKT, as this technique is called, involves visual, auditory, kinesthetic, and tactile stimulation in the learning process. Visual stimulation is that which the individual receives through the eye. Auditory stimulation is that received through the ear. Kinesthetic stimulation is that which arises in the musculature, in the tendons, and so on, as the result of body movements or tensions within the body. Tactile stimulation is that which arises in the skin from contact with outside objects.

Two special pedagogical techniques, the Fernald and the Gillingham, are often considered in the remediation of the severely retarded reader. Both approaches involve the use of as many kinds of stimulation as necessary for acquiring and retaining the ability to recognize words.

Teachers employing the Fernald approach usually begin with a tracing step. At this stage the learner listens as the teacher writes the word. The learner observes the writing, says the word as he traces (continuing until he can write the word), and says it as he writes it. As he progresses, he no longer needs the tracing, but otherwise follows the same type of procedure. Throughout the stages, words are learned as wholes, being pronounced naturally and in syllables as they are traced, studied, or written. This tracing technique is an attempt to achieve maximum stimulation for word learning.

In contrast, the Gillingham technique advocates teaching the sounds of the letters and then building these letter sounds into words, like bricks into a wall. Many educators associate this method with the familiar "phonetic" or "sound" technique. The difference lies in the fact that the Gillingham approach is based on the close association of visual, auditory, and kinesthetic elements.

Unfortunately, in some programs remedial pupils are exposed to one particular technique. The selection of the specific pedagogical procedure may depend to a large extent on the training of the clinician and the bias of the diagnostic center. Educators embrace the philosophy of individual differences, but too often accept the "one right way" of teaching reading to all retarded readers. Pupils and teachers alike have to adjust to the one procedure instead of the teacher and technique adjusting to the needs of the child. Too often, teachers have followed one policy blindly because some authority has said, "This is the way." Experience has demonstrated the fact that there is no panacea for all children. Severely retarded readers have one consistent syndrome, aside from their retardation, and that is inconsistency. The clinician must select the appropriate technique through diagnostic teaching and use all sensory pathways to reinforce the weak memory patterns. Any method or combination of methods that helps the child is the right method. A teacher must have considerable training and proficiency in all pedagogical procedures to follow this eclectic approach.

In summary, the organization of the actual remediation program can become an overwhelming barrier. The following difficulties must be overcome if an effective program is to be implemented: confusion in selecting the proper teaching environment; disagreement on the appropriate pedagogical technique; difficulty of early identification; and inadequate space, staff, and materials.

The Parent's Role

There can be no success without parental involvement and an understanding by the parent of the child's learning disability.

Parents must be notified of their responsibilities to the program. Whenever possible, special parent seminars are scheduled during the school year. Sometimes meetings are conducted by reading clinicians and/or visiting teachers trained in family life discussions. The parents have an opportunity to discuss some of the things—either old or new—that have been bothering them. Here the parents see that they are not alone; other parents share similar problems, other children have personality changes. In many cases, parents can help each other solve some of these pressing issues. The whole program is conducted in a nondirective, relaxed fashion. Psychologists are there as observers and only join in as consultants when requested to do so by the parents. The group discusses such practical problem as: How do I encourage my child to do his homework? How should I handle my child now that he is so aggressive?

At this time it might be of some value to discuss the full role of the parent.

The most powerful motivation for reading is a real desire to read. No drill can take children as far as a real interest. The kindergarten teacher stimulates this interest by telling stories, showing pictures, laughing and discussing things with children. As a pupil progresses through the grades, teachers appraise and develop his interests as part of the learning program. Parents also can do much to foster this interest.

Parents who read and enjoy reading often transmit that feeling of enjoyment to the child. Children notice that their parents talk over the problems of the day from the newspaper, laugh at funny parts of a magazine, refer to certain books for information, read interesting and exciting stories to them. In other words, the child, even before he learns to read, notes that "reading is just talk written down."

The evidence from research clearly shows that the best readers tend to be pupils whose homes are well-supplied with books, magazines, newspapers, and other reading matter, and homes in which other members of the family habitually read and enjoy it. Conversely, poor readers, other things being equal, tend to come from homes in which there is little interest or opportunity for reading. In many instances it has been found that one of the best ways to improve reading in school is to encourage it and provide for it in the home. For parents the emphasis is on encouraging, not on teaching.

The home gives the child his start in listening and speaking. Listening helps him build and store up mental images of words and to identify likenesses and differences in words. Many parents never really listen to children. Parents must encourage good listening skills and good speech patterns. A child continually hearing the word *film* pronounced *fil-um* may include the incorrect pronunciation in his oral vocabulary.

A readiness for reading is developed in the home through rich experiences that give depth and breadth to interests, normal conversations that deal with the child's experiences, broad adventures with poetry and stories, opportunities to engage in free play activities with contemporaries, and the like. The development of desirable relationships in play activities with other children should be encouraged at all times.

The ability to assume responsibility has its beginning in the home. For example, children should be taught to dress themselves and to pick up their toys, and later should be encouraged to deal with such people as the grocer and drug clerk. These are all worthwhile experiences which form the basis for later school experiences.

Many parents do not realize that one of the most common causes of reading difficulty is found in the area of personal adjustment. Reading retardation may result from an unstable emotional climate in the home. Remedial reading may not always be the answer. The child's mind simply may not be prepared for the learning experience because of other preoccupations that hold his attention. Suppose a boy's parents are quarreling seriously. This may so jeopardize his perception of affection in the home as to leave the boy feeling very insecure. He may spend a great amount of time worrying over the situation and wondering what may happen and what he can do about it. In such many situations the material presented in class just does not seem important.

Parents should be responsible for the physical welfare of their children. Every child should have a complete physical examination, including vision and hearing, before entering the first grade. Parents should not wait for a note or warning to be sent home from the school nurse.

Research and Evaluation

A great deal of research has been undertaken, and much has been written relating to the retarded reader. Unfortunately, a survey of the literature indicates that there is considerable lack of agreement among the interested professionals as to the etiology and appropriate pedagogical procedure for the dyslexic pupil. Some of the apparent barriers include the obvious lack of definitions, lack of organized programs of remediation, and invalid or unreliable measuring instruments. Even the availability of new statistical techniques and sophisticated "hardware" have not appreciably solved the problem. The old saying, "put garbage in and you get garbage out" is still applicable.

In almost all new innovative educational activities there is great difficulty in convincing people of the need for longitudinal experimental programs in which the approaches and techniques are kept pure for the length of the study. Strong efforts must be made to resist contamination with personal interpretations and biases. Dyslexia programs, if they are successful, will be at best a slow process, and only the teacher and other people who are directly involved will see the slow changes in their students' behavior. These behavioral changes are difficult to measure objectively. Consequently, the evaluation of the program should be done by the people directly involved. Unfortunately, this is sometimes impossible for local research departments to understand.

Nevertheless, it is most vital that effective longitudinal research be carried on somewhere in the country. Too often local school systems will insist on supportive research before starting a new program. I say longitudinal because the research just does not exist to show the amount of remission, the most effective teaching procedures, the optimum starting grade level, and the amount and length of therapy.

In summary, there is very limited research in the area of

the dyslexic child. Once the variables can be defined, many research and evaluation projects can be instituted to provide school systems with the most effective educational program for these disabled readers.

Summary

I do not believe that the schools will ever solve or even contain this serious problem merely through the addition of large numbers of reading specialists or diagnostic and treatment clinics. This is not to say that skilled reading clinicians are not helpful to a total reading program, only that as the educational staff becomes more sophisticated in identifying children with learning disabilities, waiting lists grow in size and the reading personnel are unable to keep pace with the overwhelming demands for their services. Special reading classes scheduled outside the regular classroom are often too large to provide effective individual remediation. Also, heavy tutorial loads cause some children to be scheduled for reading during times when classroom activities are the most interesting. Overloaded remedial or corrective classes prevent the use of reading specialists as effective resource personnel in helping teachers develop the necessary techniques and attitudes, and in assisting in the planning of effective programs for children with special reading problems.

The answer lies in developing a strong preventive, developmental, and corrective reading program in the local classroom. Administrators must make sure that they are providing the regular classroom teacher with every advantage, skill, and opportunity to do his job. Teachers must be given class sizes that are small enough to meet individual differences and techniques to adjust the pedagogic procedures to the needs of the child, not the child to the program.

EPILOGUE

This book has been written with the hope that the hundreds of thousand of families like Charles and his parents, vividly described in the prologue, will not in the future be exposed to the continuous agony of frustration and failure.

It is appropriate that medicine attempt to contribute to the educator methods of early identification; that etiological factors, once they are identified, be managed so that the learning environment of the child can be made more acceptable; that education and medicine have a basic respect for the efforts of each other, so that the child's best interests are served. *All* research must avoid the four stumbling blocks to truth:
1. The Influence of Fragile or Unworthy Authority
2. Custom
3. The Imperfection of Undisciplined Senses
4. Concealment of Ignorance by Ostentation of Seeming Wisdom

Appendices

Appendix A:
HOW PARENTS MAY CONTRIBUTE TO READING DEVELOPMENT

1. Maintain a relaxed, comfortable atmosphere at home where each child is made to feel important and wanted.

2. Give children plenty of experience—take them to the zoo, fire house, farm, historic spots, etc.

3. Be enthusiastic about school and school activities.

4. Give children a chance to talk about themselves and their interests.

5. Answer your child's questions in a simple, direct manner.

6. Praise your child for his accomplishments.

7. Develop a feeling of independence by giving him responsibility.

8. Encourage your child to associate with other children.

9. Try to interest your child in things in which he should be interested.

10. Teach your child the correct names of persons and things. Help him to associate people and places.

11. Let your child see you reading with enjoyment.

12. Provide materials similar to those in school—paste, paper, paint, scissors, etc.

13. Insist that the child know how to follow directions and pay attention.

14. Show your child that books are not the only kind of

reading. Magazines, menus, letters, road signs, etc., are other sources.

15. Follow your child's progress in school with interest but do not burden him with minute questions about his activities.

16. Provide a daily newspaper.

17. Help the child to select a good balance of educational and recreational television programs, radio programs, movies, and books.

18. Visit the school often for an objective report of your child's progress.

19. Get your child a library card and encourage him to use it.

20. Provide a quiet place for study.

21. Have periodic physical check-ups to insure that your child is in good health.

Appendix B:
JOINT ORGANIZATIONAL STATEMENT*†

The Eye and Learning Disabilities

The problem of learning disability has become a matter of increasing public concern, which has led to exploitation by some practitioners of the normal concern of parents for the

*The Executive Committees and Councils of the American Academy of Pediatrics, the American Academy of Ophthalmology and Otolaryngology, and the American Association of Ophthalmology have approved this statement.

†This statement was prepared by an ad hoc committee of the American Academy of Pediatrics, the American Academy of Ophthalmology and Otolaryngology, and the American Association of Ophthalmology, with the assistance of the president and the past president of the Division for Children with Learning Disabilities.

welfare of their children. A child's inability to read with understanding as a result of defects in processing visual symbols, a
condition which has been called dyslexia, is a major obstacle
to school learning and has far-reaching social and economic
implications. The significance and magnitude of the problem
have generated a proliferation of diagnostic and remedial procedures, many of which imply a relationship between visual
function and learning.[1]

The eye and visual training in the treatment of dyslexia
and associated disabilities have recently been reviewed† with
the following conclusions by the American Academy of Pediatrics, the American Academy of Ophthalmology and Otolaryngology, and the American Association of Ophthalmology:

1. Learning disability and dyslexia, as well as other forms
of school underachievement, require a multi-disciplinary approach from medicine, education, and psychology in diagnosis
and treatment. *Eye care should never be instituted in isolation
when a patient has a reading problem.* Children with learning
disabilities have the same incidence of ocular abnormalities,
e.g., refractive errors and muscle imbalance, as children who are
normal achievers and reading at grade level.[2,3,4] These abnormalities should be corrected.

2. Since clues in word recognition are transmitted through
the eyes to the brain, it has become common practice to at-
tribute reading difficulties to subtle ocular abnormalities pre-
sumed to cause faulty visual perception. Studies have shown
that *there is no peripheral eye defect which produces dyslexia
and associated learning disabilities.*[5,6] Eye defects do not cause
reversals of letters, words, or numbers.

3. No known scientific evidence supports claims for improving the academic abilities of learning-disabled or dyslexic children with treatment based solely on:

   a) visual training (muscle exercises, ocular pursuit,
      glasses)[7-12]
   b) neurologic organizational training (laterality training,
      balance board, perceptual training).[2-14]

Furthermore, such training has frequently resulted in unwarranted expense and has delayed proper instruction for the
child.

4. Excluding correctable ocular defects, glasses have no

value in the specific treatment of dyslexia or other learning problems. In fact, unnecessarily prescribed glasses may create a false sense of security that may delay needed treatment.

5. The teaching of learning-disabled and dyslexic children is a problem of educational science. No one approach is applicable to all children. A change in any variable may result in increased motivation of the child and reduced frustration. Parents should be made aware that mental level and psychological implications are contributing factors to a child's success or failure. Opthalmologists and other medical specialists should offer their knowledge. This may consist of the identification of specific defects, or simply early recognition. The precursors of learning disabilities can often be detected by three years of age. Since remediation may be more effective during the early years,[15] it is important for the physician to recognize the child with this problem and refer him to the appropriate service, if available, before he is of school age. Medical specialists may assist in bringing the child's potential to the best level, but the actual remedial educational procedures remain the responsibility of educators.

Glossary

Anoxia: Absence of oxygen in body tissues.

Apgar Score: A score derived by an evaluation of heart rate, color, respirations, muscle tone and reflex irritability in the newborn child. This examination is determined at one minute and again at five minutes after delivery. A low score indicates some degree of fetal distress. It is a method of quantitating the neonatal status of the newborn child.

Aphasia: Loss of speech.

Apraxia: Loss of previously acquired ability to perform intricate skilled acts.

Broca's area: The area of brain having relation to speech function.

Brodmann's area: Occipital and preoccipital areas of the brain.

Corpus callosum: Area of brain which communicates the two major hemispheres.

Diathesis: Abnormality of tissue reaction.

DNA: Carrier of genetic information.

Dysmaturity: Chronological age is not equivalent to physical age.

Electroencephalogram: Graphic record of brain waves.

Frontal lobe: The portion of the brain concerned with cognition and higher intellectual functions.

Hemianopsia: Partial loss of vision in each eye.

Humoral: Chemicals secreted by glands and carried through the blood stream for effect on peripheral functions.

Hypoxia: Deficiency of oxygen in the body.

Kinesthetic: Pertaining to muscle sense, the sense by which motion, weight, position are perceived.

Multipara: A woman who has had two or more pregnancies.

Occipital lobe: Area of brain concerned with vision.

Parietal lobe: Area of brain concerned with visual association.

Phenotype: Inherited characteristics.

Praxis: The doing or performance of action. Action by command.

Retina: The innermost tunic and perceptive structure of the eye, formed by the expansion of the optic nerve.

Thyroid: Gland that secretes the hormone that has to do with body metabolism.

Wernicke's area: The area of the brain having to do with auditory perception.

References

1. Kussmaul, A.: Disturbance of speech. In: Cyclopedia of practical medicine, 14:581–875, 1877.
2. Morgan, W. P.: A case of congenital word blindness, Brit. Med. J. 2:1378–1379, 1896.
3. Orton, S. T.: Reading, writing and speech problems in children, New York, W. W. Norton & Co., 1937.
4. Margolin, J. B., Roman, M., and Hasari, C.: Reading disability in the delinquent child: a microcosmos of psychosocial pathology. Amer. J. Orthopsychia. 25:25–35, 1955.
5. Harrower, M.: Reading failure, a warning signal, Woman's Home Companion, July, 1955, p. 43.
6. Rabinovitch, R.: Reading and learning difficulties. In: Arietti, S., Ed.: American handbook of psychiatry, Vol. 2, New York, Basic Books.
7. Critchley, M.: Developmental dyslexia, London, William Heineman Medical Books, 1964.
8. Bannatyne, A.: A suggested classification of the causes of dyslexia, Word Blind Bulletin, 1966, I, 5–13.
9. Orton, S. T., Visual functions in strephosymbolia. Arch. Ophthal. 30:707, 1943.
10. Silver, A., and Hagin, R.: Specific reading disability: an approach to diagnosis and treatment, J. Spec. Educ., 1967, 1:109–118.
11. Money, J.: The disabled reader, Baltimore, Johns Hopkins Press, 1966.

12. Rabinovitch, R.: Neurology and Psychiatry, Vol. 34, 1954, p. 363.
13. Betts, E. A.: The ABC of Language Arts Bulletin, Vol. 1, No. 4.
14. Goldberg, H. K.: The ophthalmologist looks at the reading problem, Amer. J. Ophthal., 47:67–74, 1959.
15. Brain, W. R.: Speech and handedness, Lancet 2:837, 1945.
16. Research Conference: Problems of dyslexia and related disorders. U. S. Dept. of Health, Education and Welfare, Office of Education, July 12, 1967.
17. Ertl, J. P., and Barry, W.: Researchers: quid nune I.Q.? M.D. Magazine, June 1966, p. 75.
18. Connors, C. K.: Cortically visual-evoked response in children with learning disorders. Psychophysiology, 7:418, 1970–1971.
19. Lansdell, H.: Dominance: what is it? Learning Disabilities Lecture, Johns Hopkins University, Jan. 29, 1972.
20. Schiffman, G., and Clemmens, R.: Observations on children with severe reading problems, learning disorders. Seattle, Wash., Special Child Publications, 1966.
21. Johns Hopkins Collaborative Perinatal Project. Proceedings of a Symposium: Factors affecting the growth and development of children. J. H. Press, Baltimore, 1970.
22. Castner, B. M.: Prediction of reading disability prior to first grade entrance. Amer. J. Orthopsychiat. 5:375–387, 1935.
23. DeHirsch, K.: Predicting reading failure. New York, Harper & Row, 1966.
24. Rawson, M.: Bibliography on nature, recognition and treatment of language difficulties. Orton Society, 1971.
25. Slingerland, B.: Screening test for identifying children with specific learning disabilities. Cambridge, Mass., Educators Publishing Service, 1969.
26. DeHirsch, K.: Tests designed to discover potential reading difficulties at six-year-old level. Amer. J. Orthopsychiat., 27:566–576, 1957.
27. Jansky, J. J.: American Association of Ophthalmology, Conference on Learning Disabilities, Atlantic City, N. J., June 19, 1971.
28. Meeting Street School Monograph· Early identification of children with learning disabilities. Providence, R. I., 1969.
29. Mark, H.: Brain damage in children: etiology-diagnosis-treatment. Baltimore, Williams & Wilkins.
30. WISC—Wechsler Intelligence Scale for Children. New York, The Psychological Corporation, 1949.
31. Goldberg, H. K., and Drash, P. W.: The disabled reader. J. Pediat. Ophthal., 5:11-24, 1968.
32. Koppitz, E. M.: Bender Gestalt test for young children. New York, Grune & Stratton, 1964.

33. Harris, D.: Children's drawings as measures of intellectual maturity. New York, Harcourt, Brace and World, 1963.

34. Mark, H.: Psychodiagnostics in patients with suspected minimal brain dysfunction: minimal brain dysfunction. HEW Monograph, U. S. Dept. of Health, Education and Welfare, PHS–2015, 1969.

35. Cattell, R. B.: Objective test of character-temperament. J. Gen. Psychol. 25:59–73, 1941.

36. Gesell, A.: The guidance of mental growth in infants and children. New York, MacMillan, 1931.

37. Terman, L. M., and Merrill, M. A.: Stanford-Binet Intelligence Scale: manual for the third revision form. Boston, Houghton-Mifflin, 1960.

38. Ford, F. R.: Diseases of nervous system in infancy. Springfield, Ill., Charles C Thomas, 1966.

39. Dejerine, J.: Contribution a l'étude anatamo-pathologique et clinique des differentes varietes de cecite berbale. Memoirs de la Societé de Biologie, 4:61, 1892.

40. Masland, R. L.: Brain mechanisms underlying the language function. Bull. Orton Soc., 17:1–19, 1967.

41. Strauss, A. A., and Lehtinen, L. E.: Psychopathology and education of the brain injured child. New York, Grune & Stratton, 1947.

42. Kawi, A. A., and Pasamanik, B.: Association of factors of pregnancy with the development of reading disorders in childhood. J.A.M.A., 166:1420, 1958.

43. Landau, L., and Berson, D.: Cerebral palsy and mental retardation: ocular findings. J. Pediat. Ophthal., 8:248, 1971.

44. Walsh, F. B., and Lindenberg, R.: Hypoxia in children. Bull. Johns Hopkins Hosp. 108:100–145, 1961.

45. Payne, R. S.: Minimal chronic brain syndrome in children. Develop. Med. Child Neurol. 4:21, 1962.

46. Prechtly, H., and Stemmer, C. H.: The choreiform syndrome in children. Develop. Med. Child Neurol. 4:119, 1962.

47. Werner, H., and Strauss, A.: Pathology of a figure ground relation in the child. J. Abnorm. Soc. Psychol., 36:58, 1941.

48. Critchley, M.: The problem of developmental dyslexia. Proc. Roy. Soc. Med. 56:209–212, 1963.

49. Birch, H. G., and Belmont, L.: Auditory-visual integration in normal and retarded readers. Amer. J. Orthopsychiat. 34:852–861, 1964.

50. Khoudadoust, A., Ziai, M., and Biggs, S. L.: Optic disc in normal new-borns. Amer. J. Ophthal. 66:502–504, 1968.

51. Goldberg, H. K., et al: The role of brain damage in congenital dyslexia. Amer. J. Ophthal., Vol. 50, No. 4, Oct. 1960.

52. Penfield, W., and Roberts, L.: Speech and brain-mechanisms. Princeton, New Jersey, University Press, 1959.

53. Kennard, M. A., Rabinovitch, R. D., and Wexler, D.: The abnormal electroencephalogram as related to reading disability in children with disorders of behavior. Canad. Med. Ass. J., 67: 330–333, 1952.

54. Towbin, A.: Organic causes of minimal brain dysfunction. J.A.M.A., 217:1207–1214, 1971.

55. IDEA Occasional Paper: Seminar on chemistry of learning and Memory. Yellow Springs, Ohio, Charles F. Kettering Foundation, 1970.

56. Hardy, J. B., and Peeples, M. O.: Serum bilirubin levels in newborn infants: distributions and associations with neurological abnormalities during the first year of life. Johns Hopkins Med. J. 128:265–272, 1971.

57. Birch, J. G., and Belmont, L.: Auditory-visual integration in normal and retarded readers. Amer. J. Orthopsychiat. 34:852–861, 1964.

58. Cruickshank, W. M., et. al: A teaching method for brain-injured and hyperactive children. Syracuse, Syracuse University Press, 1961.

59. Carlson, V., and Greenspoon, K.: The uses and abuses of visual training for children with perceptual-motor learning problems. Amer. J. Optom., 45:161–169, 1968.

60. Wold, R. M.: Vision and learning, the great puzzle: Parts 1, 2, 3, Optometric Weekly, Oct. 7, 14, 21, 1971.

61. Bettman, Jr., J. W., Stern, E. L., Whitsell, L. J., and Gofman, H. F.: Cerebral dominance in developmental dyslexia: role of ophthalmologist. Archiv Ophthal. 78:722–730, 1967.

62. Norn, M. S.: Rindziunskg and Skydsgaard: Ophthalmologic and orthoptic examination in dyslectics. Acta Ophthal. 47:147. 1969.

63. Blair, J., and Ryckman, D.: Visual discrimination ability among pre-readers: studies in language and language behavior. Progress Report VII, Center for Research on Language and Language Behavior, Ann Arbor, University of Michigan, 1968.

64. Piaget, J.: The origins of intelligence in children. New York, International Universities Press, 1952.

65. Koppitz: Bender.

66. Frostig, M.: An approach to the treatment of children with learning disorders, Vol. 1, Seattle, Wash., Special Child Publications, 1965.

67. Goldberg, H. K., and Guthrie, J. T.: Evaluation of visual perceptual factors in reading disability. J. Pediat. Ophthal. 9:18–25, 1972.

68. Lowder, R. G.: Perceptual ability and school achievement. Winter Haven, Fla., Winter Haven Lions Club, 1956.

69. Fernald, G.: Certain language disabilities: nature and treatment. Baltimore, William & Wilkins, 1943.

70. Masland, R.: Review of studies relating to visual motor and visual perceptual training. Speech at Montgomery County Health Dept., April 1968.

71. Johnson, D., and Myklebust, H.: Learning disabilities: educational principals and practices. New York, Grune & Stratton, 1967.

72. Ford, M.: Auditory-visual and tactual-visual integration in relation to reading ability. Perceptual Motor Skills, 24:831–841, 1967.

73. Hardy, W. J., and Bordley, J.: Hearing evaluation in children. Otolaryng. Clin. N. Amer., Feb. 1969, pp. 3–26.

74. Cherry, E. C.: Some experiments on the recognition of speech. J. Acoust. Soc. Amer. 25:975, 1953.

75. Thompson, B. B.: A longitudinal study of auditory discrimination. J. Ed. Res., 56:376, 1963.

76. Liberman, A. M., Cooper, F. S., et al.: Perception of the speech code. Psychol. Rev. 74:431–461, Nov. 1967.

77. Wepman, J. M.: Dyslexia: its relationship to language acquisition and concept formation. In: Money, J., Ed.: Reading disability. Baltimore, Johns Hopkins Press, 1962.

78. Witkin, B. R.: Auditory perception: implications for language development. J. Res. Devel. in Educ., College of Education, University of Georgia, Vol. 3, No. 1, 1969, pp. 53–71.

79. Bryant and Patterson: Reading disability.

80. Denhoff, E.: Learning disorders in children. Ross Laboratories Report, Columbus, Ohio, p. 37.

81. Bender, L.: Psychopathology of children with organic brain disorders. Springfield, Ill., Charles C Thomas, 1956.

82. Bakwin, H., and Bakwin, R. M.: Clinical management of behavior disorders in children, 2nd Ed. Philadelphia, W. B. Saunders, 1960.

83. Kanner, L.: Child psychiatry, 2nd Ed. Springfield, Ill., Charles C Thomas, 1948, p. 542.

84. Hess, R. D.: Maternal behavior and the development of reading readiness in urban negro children. Paper prepared for the Claremont Reading Conference, Claremont, California, Feb. 10, 1968, p. 15.

85. Spielberger, D. D.: Anxiety and behavior. New York, Academic Press, 1966.

86. Diethelm, O., and Jones, M. R.: Influence of anxiety on atten-

tion, learning, retention and thinking. Arch. Neurol. Psychiat., 58:325–326, 1947.

87. Harrower, M.: Reading failure.
    Home Companion July 1955, p. 43.

88. Dygert, J. H.: (Quoted in) "We must give jobs to school drop-outs." Parade, 8:29, 1971, p. 23.

89. Ingram, T. T. S., and Reid, J. F.: Developmental aphasia observed in a department of child psychiatry. Arch. Dis. Child. 31:161–172, 1956.

90. Fabian, A. A.: Clinical and experimental studies of school children who are retarded in reading. Quart. J. Child Behav. 3:15, 1951.

91. Blanchard, P.: Psychogenic factors in some cases of reading disability. Amer. J. Orthopsychiat. 5:361–374, 1935.

92. Missildine, W. H.: The emotional background of thirty children with reading disability with emphasis on its coercive elements. Nerv. Child 5:263–272, 1946.

93. Kanner, L., and Eisenberg, L.: Childhood problems in relation to the family. Pediatrics 20:155–164, 1957.

94. Trevor-Roper, P.: Evolution of the dominant eye. Insight, Vol. 5, No. 10, Nov. 1970.

95. Subirana, A.: The problem of cerebral dominance: the relationship between handedness and language function. Logos 4:85, 1961.

96. Gordon, H.: Left-handedness and mirror writing, especially among defective children. Brain, 43:313, 1921.

97. Subirana, A.: The relationship between handedness an dlanguage function. Int. J. Neurol. 4:215–234, 1964.

98. Subirana: Problem of cerebral dominance.

99. Benton, A. L.: The problem of cerebral dominance. Bull. Orton Soc. 16:38–53, 1966.

100. Mountcastle, V. B., Ed.: Interhemispheric relations and cerebral dominance. Baltimore, Johns Hopkins Press, 1962, pp. 117–129.

101. Sperry, R. W.: The great cerebral commissure. Scientific American, Jan. 1926, pp. 42–52.

102. Penfield, W., and Roberts, L.: Speech and brain mechanisms. Princeton, New Jersey, Princeton University Press, 1959.

103. Rasmussen, A. T.: Lateralization of cerebral speech dominance. J. Neurosurg. 23:400, 1964.

104. Critchley: Problem.

105. Brain: Speech.

106. Subirana: Problem of cerebral dominance.

107. Orton, S. T.: Reading, writing and speech problems in children. London, Chapman & Hall, 1937.

108. Brain: Speech.
109. Zangwill, O. L.: Dyslexia in relation to cerebral dominance, reading disability. Baltimore, Johns Hopkins Press, pp. 103–113.
110. Zangwill: Dyslexia.
111. Whittey, P. A., and Kopel, D. D.: Factors associated with the etiology of reading disability. J. Educ. Res. 29:449–459, 1936.
112. Johnston, P. W.: The relation of certain anomalies of vision in lateral dominance to reading disability. Monograph for the Society for Research and Child Development, Vol. 71, No. 2, Washington, D. C., 1942.
113. Smith, L.: A study of laterality characteristics of retarded readers and reading achievers. J. Exp. Res. 18:321–329, 1950.
114. Hermelin, B., and O'Connor, N.: Right and left handed reading of braille. Nature 231:470, 1971.
115. Benton, C. D., and McCann, J. W.: Dyslexia and dominance. J. Ped. Ophthal., 6:220, 1969.
116. Berner, G. E., and Berner, D. E.: Relation of ocular dominance, handedness, and the controlling eye in binocular vision. Arch. Ophthal. 50:603–608, 1953.
117. Orton: Reading (see Ref. 3).
118. Clifford, J. K.: Stop the reading disability frauds. Optometric Weekly, July, 1961.
119. Critchley: Problem.
120. Bryant, N. D., and Patterson, R. R.: Reading Disability: part of a syndrome of neurological functioning. Paper presented at International Reading Association, 1962.
121. Hallgren, B.: Specific dyslexia (congenital word blindness), a clinical and genetic study. Acta Psychiat. Neurol., suppl. 65, 1950.
122. Childs, B.: Biological basis of human behavior. California Institute of Technology, March 16, 1964.
123. Silver, A. A., and Hagin, R. A.: Specific reading disability: follow-up studies. Amer. J. Orthopsychiat. 34:95–102, 1964.
124. Bryant and Patterson: Reading disability.
125. Boder, E.: Developmental dyslexia, a diagnostic screening procedure based on characteristic patterns of reading and spelling. Claremont Reading Conference, 32nd Yearbook, 1968, p. 173.
126. Ingram, T. T. S.: Pediatric aspects of specific developmental dysphasia, dyslexia, and dysgraphia. Cereb. Palsy Bull. 2:254–277, 1960.
127. Critchley: Problem.
128. Hallgren: Specific dyslexia.
129. Hermann, K.: Reading disability: a medical study of word

blindness and related handicaps. Springfield, Ill., Charles C Thomas, 1959.

130. Rawson, M. B.: Developmental language disability: adult accomplishments of dyslexic boys. Baltimore, Johns Hopkins Press, 1968. See No. 24.

131. Agranoff, B.: The chemistry of learning. An IDEA Occasional paper, Yellow Springs, Ohio, C. F. Kettering Research Lab.

Index